Praise for
*Heal Your Hormones, Reclaim Yourself*

*"Dr. Sonya Jensen has taken the complex world of female biology and translated it into something deeply human, intimate, and profoundly healing. Reading this book feels like sitting across from a wise friend who sees you, truly sees you, and hands you the tools to remember your power. Sonya has created a map for women to move through chaos with compassion, to release shame, and to rediscover the brilliance that's been there all along."*

— **Dr. Mindy Pelz**, *New York Times* best-selling author of *Fast Like a Girl*, *Eat Like a Girl*, and *Age Like a Girl*

*"This book is a powerful guide that helps women understand the deep connection between their hormones, emotions, and past experiences. I recommend it because it gives women the tools needed to release their old patterns keeping them stuck. Once you break free, you also reclaim your health and step into your most authentic self, which we all deserve!"*

— **Dr. Caitlin Czezowski, DC, CFMP, CACCP**, a.k.a. @doc.talks.detox

*"Dr. Sonya Jensen's* Heal Your Hormones, Reclaim Yourself *is a grounded, bio-individual guide that meets women where they are body, mind, and spirit. Dr. Jensen reminds us that healing isn't linear and invites readers to break generational patterns with practical tools for nervous system regulation, reflection, and daily self-care. Most importantly, she helps women integrate their own innate wisdom into their healing with evidence-informed strategies, so progress feels personal, sustainable, and deeply empowering. This is a thoughtfully crafted resource for all women."*

— **Cynthia Thurlow, NP**, best-selling author of *Intermittent Fasting for Women* and TEDx speaker

*"Dr. Sonya Jensen helps me stay balanced and happy in my body. Her approach is so multi-dimensional—feminine, Western, Eastern, lab work, inner work—the lived wisdom that comes from knowing how women heal best. She's so solid, and I'm so grateful."*

— **Danielle LaPorte**, founder of the Centered App

*"Dr. Sonya Jensen's revolutionary HER Method brilliantly connects our hormonal symptoms not just to our emotions and relationships, but to the generational stories we carry in our cells. This is the essential guide for any woman ready to stop managing symptoms, trust her body's deep intelligence, and begin the journey of true healing. She blends Ayurveda, yoga poses, thoughtful meditations, and encouraging words, making you feel like you are just sharing a cup of tea with your sister. This fusion of Eastern and Western medicine, and integrative medicine and psychology, is a unique and needed approach to hormone imbalances. I wish I would have had something like this in my early years as a traditionally trained OB-GYN treating women."*

— **Dr. Tara Scott**, OB-GYN

*"I have the privilege of knowing Dr. Sonya Jensen as both a trusted colleague and a dear friend, and I deeply admire the clarity and care she brings to her work. In this book, she delivers a refreshing, empowering perspective on hormone health—one rooted in personalization, compassion, and clinical excellence. Her guidance will inspire readers to approach their hormones with curiosity, respect, and confidence."*

— **Dr. Nasha Winters, ND, FABNO**, author of *The Metabolic Approach to Cancer*

*"Dr. Sonya Jensen has written a truly beautiful and much-needed book that reframes hormonal chaos through the lens of the mental and emotional load so many women carry. Her HER Method helps women recognize how overdrive, people-pleasing, and perfectionism show up not only in our lives but also in our hormones. This is the compassionate, grounded guide every woman deserves."*

— **Carrie Jones, ND, FABNE, MPH, MSCP**

*"Dr. Sonya bridges science and soul in a way every woman's body has been waiting for.* Heal Your Hormones, Reclaim Yourself *is a road map back to connection. A reminder that your body isn't broken, it's breaking open. Your hormones speak the language of your body, whispering through signals and symptoms, guiding you back to alignment. This book feels like coming home to yourself."*

— **Dr. Melissa Sonners**, author of *The Connection Code*,
nervous system & brainwave regulation guide

# Heal Your Hormones, Reclaim Yourself

# Heal Your Hormones, Reclaim Yourself

Connect the Dots Between **Hormonal Chaos, Emotional Overload,** and **Relationship Pain** with the **HER Method**

DR. SONYA JENSEN, ND

HAY HOUSE

**HAY HOUSE INDIA**
New Delhi • London • Sydney
Carlsbad, California • New York City

**Hay House Publishers (India) Pvt Ltd**
Muskaan Complex, Plot No. 3, B-2, Vasant Kunj, New Delhi – 110070, India

Hay House LLC, P.O. Box 5100, Carlsbad, CA 92018-5100, USA
Hay House UK Ltd, 1st Floor, Crawford Corner, 91-93 Baker Street, London W1U 6QQ, UK
Hay House Australia Publishing Pty Ltd, 18/36 Ralph St., Alexandria NSW 2015, Australia

Email: contact@hayhouse.co.in
Website: www.hayhouse.co.in

*Indexer:* J S Editorial, LLC
*Cover design:* Jordan Wannemacher
*Interior design:* Julie Davison
*Interior photos/illustrations:* Madushani



First published by Hay House India, 2026
10 9 8 7 6 5 4 3 2 1

ISBN 978-93-6611-516-0

Printed at Repro India Limited

MIX
Paper from responsible sources
FSC® C047271

Hay House is committed to a sustainable future for our business, our readers and our planet. This book is made from Forest Stewardship Council® certified paper.

*To my nieces,*
*Armelle, Seva, Xari, London, and Jazy,*
*I hope you realize the power you*
*have and the wisdom you carry.*

# CONTENTS

## Part II:

### The HER Method—A Proven Method to Heal Hormonal Chaos and Emotional Overload

# Foreword

There are moments in life when a book comes along that doesn't just inform, it transforms. *Heal Your Hormones, Reclaim Yourself* is one of those rare books.

Dr. Sonya Jensen has written a body of work that every woman deserves to read. She has taken the complex world of female biology and translated it into something deeply human, intimate, and profoundly healing. With her signature blend of science, soul, and story, Sonya weaves a narrative that makes hormones, so often misunderstood, feared, or dismissed, feel like the sacred messengers they truly are.

Her HER Method, connecting hormones, emotions, and relationships, illuminates a truth I've witnessed in millions of women: You cannot heal your body without also healing the woman living inside it. We've been taught to separate our biology from our emotions, to chase "balance" through control and suppression. Sonya invites us instead to listen. To understand that our hormones are not the enemy, but the language of our inner wisdom—guiding us through every season of womanhood with insight and grace.

What moves me most about this pivotal book is that it comes from lived experience. Sonya doesn't just teach the science of hormones; she embodies the journey of healing. Her personal stories are honest and raw, filled with the same vulnerability that so many women feel but rarely speak aloud. That's why her words will reach you on a cellular level. They remind you that your symptoms are not a flaw to fix—they are communication from your body, calling you home to yourself.

Reading this book feels like sitting across from a wise friend who sees you, truly sees you, and hands you the tools to remember your power. Sonya has created a map for women to move through chaos with compassion, to release shame, and to rediscover the brilliance that's been there all along.

This is more than a book about hormones—it's a reclamation. A call to remember that you are cyclical, intuitive, and powerful beyond measure. Whether you are navigating your first period, motherhood, perimenopause, or the deep wisdom of postmenopause, Sonya's guidance meets you exactly where you are and walks beside you toward healing.

I am honored to call Dr. Sonya Jensen a colleague, and even more honored to call her my dear friend. Her work reflects the kind of inner medicine the world needs most right now, medicine that honors both the science and the spirit of being a woman.

May *Heal Your Hormones, Reclaim Yourself* be the guide that leads you back to your truth, your vitality, and the woman you were always meant to be.

**— Dr. Mindy Pelz, DC**

*New York Times* best-selling author of *Fast Like a Girl, Eat Like a Girl* and *Age Like a Girl*

# Acknowledgments

I didn't always know that I would be an author and still find myself in awe of how all this came to be. Sharing your innermost thoughts and ideas with the world feels like such a vulnerable and scary act at times. It is through the encouragement and support of so many in my life that I have been able to bring this book to the world. Especially from my husband, Nick Jensen, and my two boys, Kaiyn and Soryn. Thank you for creating space for me and constantly reminding me that what I have to say is important. Your unconditional love and willingness to adjust our lives so I could write this book means the world to me. Thank you for always making me laugh, for holding me when I cried, and for teaching me the beauty and various depths of relationships so I could share that with the world through these words.

Being able to speak and share my ideas as a woman is important to me on so many levels. Most importantly to break the cycle of generational silence and to stop the habit of hiding that many women find themselves in. I am so grateful to my nani, Amarjit Kaur Chohan, a woman who even in her hiding of herself and in the suffering from her trauma was able to model a life filled with love and with a capacity to find joy from the small things in her world and the relationships she held close. Her wisdom, her strength, and the nurturing she modeled for me is what inspired me to continually look at all the angles of any story that women carry with them, which is the foundation of this book. I miss her every day and hope these words and this desire to support women everywhere honors their stories and honors her memory.

It is from the willingness of my patients and the women in my life to share themselves with me, their raw, messy, and beautiful truths, that I was able to write this book. I am so thankful for all of you for sharing your heart, your challenges, and your dreams and for putting your trust in me to help you. It is what allowed me to bring this work to the world. You have inspired me with your courage as you brave your way through the chaos of life.

It takes so much care and love to birth a book. I am so grateful to Patty Gift and the Hay House team for their support and for believing in this work enough to take me on as an author. Your encouraging words and ability to see the author in me gave me the courage needed to bring these words onto paper for the world to read. Thank you, Anne Barthel, my editor, for the insightful conversations and for making me feel at home and helping me stay grounded in the process. Your caring and supportive approach helped ease my anxiety and self-doubt, which allowed me to work on this book from a place of ease.

Sometimes when you don't believe in yourself, you can hold on to the belief others have in you to keep going. I want to thank Stephanie Tade, my agent, for reminding me that I belong here. That I belong in the seat of an author next to the authors that I admire and have learned so much from over the years. To my soul sisters Dr. Mindy Pelz, Dr. Melissa Sonners, Melissa Alonso, Andrea Siebert, Dr. Caitlin Czezowski, Jacqueline Wener, and Rozeela Nand, thank you for continuously speaking words of encouragement and guiding me along the way when there were times I wanted to hide under a rock. To my life sisters, Kristen Rich and Hasina Masood, thank you for the school pickups so I could write even an hour longer and for the daily support in raising our boys. To my family—in-laws, aunts, uncles, brother, brothers- and sisters-in-law, cousins, and all—thank you for all the support you have given me; it is the foundation that I land on and the comfort I rely on. Learning from these relationships and walking this life with you all helps me understand the power of community and the impact it has on a woman's health.

To my sister and best friend, Sophia Sandhu, thank you for being the sounding board I needed to keep on the path of writing from my heart. To my parents, Gurjit Singh Grewal and Manmohan Kaur Grewal, for making the sacrifice of leaving their home in India so we could live out our dreams, and for teaching me the meaning of resilience and tenacity when it comes to going after what you want but also the meaning of true *seva*, service to the world. It is that desire to serve that helped me complete this book in the midst of my own beautifully chaotic life.

# Introduction

You are not broken. You might feel lost, as though your emotions are all over the place. Your body may be changing in ways you don't understand—your hormones going up, down, and sideways—leaving you feeling disconnected and out of control. Your relationships may be challenging you in ways you never thought possible, testing your patience and your resilience. And yet, amid all that change and chaos, a deep inner strength waits—not lost, just buried—ready for you to remember her.

Healing is not linear, nor is it tidy. It's messy, raw, and often overwhelming—especially when your healing doesn't just impact you but everyone around you.

This journey can feel especially daunting when life keeps demanding you to show up every day: at work, as a mom, a wife, a daughter, a friend. The external expectations seem endless, often piling on while you're already navigating the internal whirlwind of hormonal shifts, emotional turbulence, and physical discomfort. But this book is here to remind you that you don't have to navigate this alone. Your hormones and emotions are not working against you—they are trying to communicate with you, to guide you back to balance.

Over the years, I've worked with women of all ages and stages—teenagers making decisions about birth control, young women grappling with fertility struggles, and mothers battling fatigue and burnout. I've seen women who have turned to the medical system, only to be told that "nothing is wrong," even as they struggle to move through their day. They fight to keep the weight off, to focus through the brain fog, to understand why they feel emotionally fragile, and to manage the strain their hormones and emotions place on their most important relationships.

The truth is, your hormones are deeply intertwined with your emotions, your relationships, and your overall sense of self. When your hormones are imbalanced, it's not just your body that feels it—your emotions can feel heightened, your patience tested, and your ability to connect with others strained. These interconnected systems—your hormones, emotions, and relationships—are all calling for your attention, not to overwhelm you but to guide you toward healing and deeper connection with yourself and the people you love. This book is your companion for that journey, helping you untangle the chaos and find clarity, strength, and balance within.

Throughout this book, I will share stories from women I've had the privilege of working with. These stories are not just examples—they're reflections of a greater collective experience. They offer insight into what I call the **HER Cycle**, where your hormones, emotions, and relationships meet.

## The Path That Chose Me

It is my own hormonal journey that has fueled my passion and commitment to understanding the deeper "why" behind a woman's discomforts. While my background in cell and molecular biology, paired with my training as a naturopathic doctor, provided me with a solid foundation in understanding the human body, the science of its systems, and the therapeutic modalities that support healing—such as herbal medicine, traditional Chinese medicine, nutrition, hormone replacement therapy, and intravenous therapies—it was my personal healing journey that opened my eyes to something much deeper. It invited me to explore the intricate and often overlooked connection between the emotional body, the soul body, and the physical body, and how this connection profoundly impacts hormonal health.

Through training as a yoga teacher and diving into the shamanic medicine wheel, I began to see myself—and my story—through a new lens. These practices allowed me to uncover layers of my identity, my traumas, and the subconscious beliefs that were directly influencing my hormones. I discovered how unhealed trauma, deeply embedded in the body, was silently altering my hormonal balance and, as a result, affecting my relationships, my emotions, and my ability to thrive. The journey revealed to me how much we carry—physically, emotionally, and spiritually—and how the burdens of unprocessed pain and stress show up as symptoms in our bodies.

As I peeled back those layers, it became clear that my healing was also pointing me toward something greater—a deeper purpose. I didn't always envision myself doing this work. At various points, I dreamed of becoming a pediatric occupational therapist, a criminal psychologist, or even a dancer and choreographer. But life had other plans. The universe kept nudging me toward this path—one that required me to confront my inner child, explore ancestral trauma, and untangle the subconscious beliefs that shaped how I saw myself and my body. I began to see that supporting women wasn't just something I could do—it was something I had to do.

These experiences and insights have been the catalyst for my work and my desire to help other women not only understand their hormonal health but also uncover their stories, beliefs, and experiences that may be keeping them stuck in cycles of imbalance. Healing the physical body is only one part of the journey. True healing requires us to address the emotional and spiritual layers that are intricately tied to our hormones and our relationships, allowing us to reclaim the vibrant, whole version of ourselves that may have felt lost along the way. This book is a reflection of that discovery and an invitation for you to explore these connections in your own life.

## Changing the Story

I've always felt a deep pull to fight against the injustices faced by women and children, but it wasn't until I explored my own trauma and relationship with my body that I understood why. Women are the first relationship every human being experiences. To support women is to support humanity. When a woman heals, she doesn't heal alone—she heals forward and backward, through generations.

But healing becomes difficult in a world that rarely teaches us to value ourselves beyond our appearance. From a young age, many of us are taught that our worth lies in how we look—and how well we can maintain that image. We're not taught how to care for our bodies as they change, or how to honor the natural rhythms that shape us. So when we begin to age and move through perimenopause and menopause, many women feel invisible—pushed aside by a culture that prizes youth over wisdom. But the truth is, this phase of life is not a decline. It's a powerful initiation into a deeper, wiser version of yourself.

How did we get here? Why aren't we having more conversations about the profound physical, emotional, social, and relational changes women experience throughout life?

These are questions we must ask as a collective—but also as individuals. And they are questions I hope you'll sit with as you move through the pages of this book.

Over the years of working with women, I've come to understand that I could only take my patients as far in their healing as I had gone in my own. Speaking to women about their relationship with food meant confronting my own history with anorexia. Helping women with polycystic ovarian syndrome (PCOS) required me to explore the roots of my own ovarian cysts and the lifestyle and emotional patterns contributing to them. Supporting women through painful, heavy periods meant facing the emotional trauma I had long stored in my reproductive system due to sexual abuse. To help them change their story, I had to be willing to rewrite my own.

Through years of research and introspection, I deepened my understanding of hormones, the body-mind connection, and how adverse childhood experiences alter stress adaptation and increase inflammation. As I pieced these insights together in my own healing journey, I found myself better equipped to guide others. Over time, my practice became a space where women healed from conditions they once believed were beyond hope. Women who had been told they could never have children were getting pregnant. Those diagnosed with chronic thyroid conditions and told they'd need medication for life were thriving without it. Women facing hysterectomies due to fibroids were not only shrinking their fibroids but fully healing their hormones.

These women took their power back—they were no longer victims of their circumstances or changing bodies, but fully in charge of their healing and deeply connected to themselves. I could help them do this because I had finally committed to healing myself. My hope as you read this book is that you, too, begin to see yourself in the stories of these women and the triumph they feel when they get to know their truth and realize that healing is possible. When everything you do and see is through the lens of your emotions and those emotions are being influenced by your always-changing hormones, it is easy to feel lost and think that this feeling or condition will always be a part of your life. But when you begin to unravel the cycle, when you learn how to support your hormones, feel grounded in your body, and steady in your emotions, you begin to experience a freedom that touches every part of your life. You become more present in your relationships, more connected to your purpose, and more able to thrive.

That's the world I dream of: a world where women can be in spaces of deep love and acceptance, where they are seen, heard, and honored exactly as they are. A world where we can share the highs, the lows, and the stories that leave us breathless or hopeless—and feel held in that sharing. When you lose hope—when a doctor tells you that the only solution is a pill, that your eggs are dwindling, or that your symptoms are all in your head—it's easy to feel trapped. Trapped in a body that feels like it's betraying you, leaving you frustrated with the very vessel that allows this human experience.

And yet, even in that loneliness, you are never truly alone. There is an unbreakable thread that weaves through every woman, connecting her to those who came before, those beside her now, and those yet to come. That thread is sacred. And while every woman's story is different, many of the root struggles are the same: We have not been given the time, space, or support to fully heal, but that time is now.

## What to Expect

Part I of this book will give you clues to the why behind your symptoms, diagnosis, or disconnect in your relationships. It will wake up questions and curiosities about your own story. It will give you a glimpse into the science of that story and its connection to your hormonal health and the health of your relationships. You will be able to identify the connection between the various hormones that govern your reproductive health and the neurotransmitters that govern your emotions, all the while understanding the environmental influences that impact how they function. You will learn the Hierarchy of Hormonal Healing, a system that breaks down the sequence of healing, and the modalities and support that will help you heal. You will have an opportunity to find your hormonal identity, an identity that reflects the health of your hormones through a quiz that will give you insight into how *your* body reacts to stress. This self-discovery through self-awareness and self-curiosity will help you become aware of your thought patterns, aware of the armor you have on, aware of the personalities you have had to create to fit in, belong, and feel safe, and aware of the million little choices you have made throughout your life that influenced your health.

Part II is where knowledge becomes action. This is where I introduce you to the **HER Method**—a practical and powerful approach to help you reconnect with your body, regulate your hormones, and reclaim your well-being. In my years of work, I noticed patterns emerging. Women would arrive in my office, not only seeking relief from symptoms like weight gain, brain fog, or fatigue, but yearning for something deeper—a connection to themselves. Their hormonal imbalances weren't just biological; they were interwoven with their emotions, environments, and relationships. This realization led me to develop the **HER Method**, which explores the dynamic relationship between **Hormones**, **Emotions**, and **Relationships** to empower women to create lasting health and harmony in all aspects of their lives.

The HER Method gives you a proven system with steps to understanding what your body needs to heal. What tests you need to understand your hormones, what foods and exercise are best suited for your hormone identity and blueprint.

The HER Method is not just about healing; it's about awakening—to your strength, your story, and the vibrant potential that is uniquely yours to embrace through simple tools you can incorporate right away.

For young women in their reproductive years, my hope is that this book becomes a guide to empowerment—supporting you in making informed, aligned decisions for your body and your future.

For women in perimenopause or menopause, navigating the shifting landscape of body and mind, I hope these pages reflect the depth and wisdom of your lived experience. It may stir reflections on choices you've made, but more importantly, it will offer you the tools, understanding, and clarity to move forward with compassion and strength as you write this next chapter of your life.

It's time to connect the dots and recognize the immense power of your story and how it has shaped your life. It's time to understand your hormones, embrace your emotions, and elevate your relationships. This is where the healing begins.

PART I

# The Invisible Link

## What Your Hormones Are Really Trying to Tell You

CHAPTER 1

# Why Am I Falling Apart?

*"You saved my life."*

I wasn't expecting to hear that from my first patient of the day—especially on a day when I felt exhausted and wasn't even sure how I had made it into the office. That day, I found myself questioning whether my work as a naturopathic doctor truly made a difference, reflecting on the many women I'd seen over the years and wondering if it was enough. "If I hadn't reached out to you, I don't know if I'd still be here," she continued. "I was told the only way out of this depression was medication, but the last time I took it, everything got worse." I could see her eyes fill with tears, and I struggled to hold back mine. I understood that feeling all too well—the weight of trying to keep going despite the emotional and physical challenges. My life is beautiful, and I am deeply grateful for it, yet I, too, sometimes battle with my emotions, my body, and the chaos of life. This struggle is what keeps me grounded in the work I do with women. Moments like this remind me that my efforts to maintain my own emotional and hormonal well-being aren't just for me—they're for every woman who sits across from me.

"I was starting to hate my life, even myself," she said. "The stress of my husband's illness, my teenage daughter, and a full-time job left me feeling hopeless and drained. I didn't know there was another way, and I'm so thankful for you. You gave me hope, a place to share my pain, and another chance for me and my family." At that point, I couldn't hold back the tears any longer.

Every time I feel drained or ready for a break, the universe reminds me why I do this work. Through the stories of women who trust me with their struggles, I see the profound impact of our thoughts, actions, and presence. These moments reinforce the responsibility, and the privilege I have, to be part of their journey. Because the truth is, even a small choice or shift in perspective can change someone's life and ripple out to those around them.

This is why your decision to pick up this book and prioritize your health is so powerful. Choosing yourself isn't selfish—it's essential. When you take steps to heal what's not working, you create space for growth, not just for you but for everyone in your orbit. The ripple effect is real; it could even save a life.

We've all been where my patient was—sitting in the chaos of life, frozen in overwhelm. Kids running wild, a boss piling on demands, a partner needing help, the dog barking for attention, deadlines looming—all while your inner world screams for relief. That external chaos doesn't stay outside; it impacts your inner world, especially your hormones. Yet, we often don't see the connection until something stops us—a diagnosis, a loss, or rock bottom.

Every woman that has walked into my office seeking help for her hormones begins to realize very quickly that there is more to her symptoms. She may come in hoping for a quick fix but over time realizes that the hormonal symptoms she has are not the cause of her suffering but a result of multiple layers of stress and her own unique story. What has become very clear over the years of working with these women but is not well understood in the medical community is that you cannot separate mental health from your hormonal health.

Imagine your body as a symphony orchestra. Your hormones are the musicians, and your mental health is the melody they create together. When each instrument plays in harmony, the music flows beautifully—your emotions feel balanced, your thoughts are clear, and your sense of well-being is steady. But if even one musician is out of tune or playing off beat, it disrupts the entire symphony. Hormonal health and mental health are deeply intertwined, much like the musicians and the melody. You can't fully enjoy or fix the melody without addressing the instruments creating it. Similarly, you can't separate your emotional well-being from the hormonal balance in your body. When one is off, the other feels the impact, and it's only by working with both that you can restore harmony and balance.

Understanding the connection between hormone health and mental health is not just vital for wellness—it's lifesaving. Approximately 5 to 8 percent of women experience premenstrual dysphoric disorder (PMDD), a severe form of premenstrual syndrome (PMS) linked to significant mood changes, depression, and even suicidal thoughts. During perimenopause, women are two to three times more likely to experience major depression, and the suicide risk escalates, making this transitional phase critical for mental health intervention. These statistics underscore the importance of addressing how hormones influence emotions, thoughts, and behaviors. Without understanding this interplay, women can feel trapped in cycles of stress and emotional overwhelm, unaware of the biological factors contributing to their struggles. By learning about these connections, women can take steps to heal holistically, breaking cycles of hormonal imbalance and emotional distress. This book bridges the gap between how you feel and how your hormones function, offering tools and insights that empower you to take control of your health and reduce the risks of mental health crises.

Stress in all its forms is the key driving force toward imbalance, especially when we don't understand it and what it is trying to tell us. How you manage stress and how your hormones react to it affect everything: your body, mind, emotions, and relationships; and the stress begins talking to you through your symptoms. In my practice, I've witnessed incredible transformations when women finally listen to their bodies and the stories they're telling. Your body whispers through symptoms like insomnia, brain fog, low libido, irritability, fatigue, or weight gain. Ignore those whispers, and they'll get louder until you're forced to pay attention. Your body holds wisdom and love for you. It speaks so you can reconnect with the powerful woman you are underneath the noise. When you finally listen, that's when true healing begins.

## Cycle of Hormonal Chaos

You are a force holding everything together, the woman who shows up day after day with strength and grace. But beneath that exterior, I know there's a part of you that feels frayed—a quiet pain that surfaces when the world stops watching. The sadness, doubt, and mental chaos can feel overwhelming when you don't understand the why behind it. No one prepared you for the emotional and physical shifts you'd face as life unfolded, from the subtle whispers of your ancestry that influence your cells and your biology to the relentless demands of everyday life, shaping your emotions, hormones, and relationships.

Each phase of life—puberty, the time you felt those newly formed curves and the swelling of your breasts, the reproductive years where you felt the rhythm of your monthly cycles and maybe even pregnancy, perimenopause (or "reverse puberty," or the era of "hormonal chaos"), and finally the transition into menopause, the Wise Woman Phase—carries with it profound hormonal and emotional shifts. These seasons of change often leave a woman feeling misunderstood and feeling like she's falling apart and broken. Yet, this journey is not one of flaws but of transformation—a process shaped by history, habits, and the layers of your personal HERstory. What's critical to remember is that these experiences through the phases hold the keys to your healing, not your undoing.

You may feel unmoored, your emotions spiraling, your body shifting in unfamiliar ways as your hormones fluctuate, and your relationships testing you in ways you never anticipated. Amid this change, in the eye of this storm, lies something unshakable—a stillness, a strength that has always been within you.

This is your **HER Wisdom**—your innate intelligence, a deep knowing imprinted in every cell of your body. It's not something you've lost; it's something waiting patiently beneath the noise of life. It's your quiet power, ready for you to recognize and reclaim. This is your moment—your moment to realize that the chaos doesn't define you. You are whole, and through understanding yourself and your hormones more deeply, you can rise into the fullness of who you are.

Your hormones are like messengers, constantly communicating with your body in response to the choices you make, the stories you carry, and the environment around you. When you don't prioritize sleep, overindulge in processed foods, push through every demand without setting boundaries, or rush through your day, you're sending signals to your hormones that you're in survival mode. This creates a cascade of stress messages to your cells, leaving you exhausted, foggy, and irritable—and let's face it, maybe even unfairly blaming your loved ones for how you feel.

Understanding how your hormones influence your emotions, mental health, and relationships is the first step to reclaiming balance and yourself. They orchestrate everything from your energy to your mood, so when you're stuck in chronic stress, it's no wonder you feel off. Healing starts with this awareness, recognizing how your daily habits influence this intricate hormonal dance, and learning to choose behaviors that tell your body it's safe to heal, thrive, and feel good again.

So, what exactly is your **HERstory**, and how does it impact your hormones? You may think you've forged your own way, but the truth is, your story connects back to those of the women before you. Their stories are passed down through your biology and through your choices and through your hormones. The story of people-pleasing, sacrificing your own happiness for others, and silencing your voice that eventually becomes a belief, passed down through generations. That belief then shapes your identity, influencing your hormones and behaviors, which in turn reinforces the very belief that shapes the health of your hormones, emotions, and relationships. You may find, as you start to discover what your story is, that you've been in a storyline not of your choosing but one laid out by family expectations or the larger narrative society has given women for generations or even the stresses and traumas your ancestors carried. We will dive deeply into understanding the connection between generational stress and trauma and the stories you may be telling yourself, and how they impact the health of your hormones—and then how you can change and heal those stories to heal your body. The moment you begin to work with your body, your body begins to work for you. The moment you ask yourself the question, *Where did this story come from?* you begin to create an opportunity to change the trajectory of your hormonal, emotional, and relational health.

## Breaking the Illusion of "I'm Fine"

Women have spent years not feeling heard by their doctors. A patient once shared with me, "I went to my doctor and told him I feel anxious for no reason, I can't sleep, I'm gaining weight, my joints are achy, and all he said to me was, 'Your labs are normal—it's just part of aging.'" Essentially, she was being told it was all in her head. But here's the truth: Your body doesn't lie.

It has taken decades for the medical community to finally begin recognizing the importance of understanding a woman's hormonal journey and its profound impact on every aspect of her health, especially her mental health. When your hormones are changing, so is your ability to adapt to or respond to stress. When your body speaks to you—through symptoms like skin issues, heavy or painful bleeding, or exhaustion—it's telling a story. It's a cry for help.

Often, these symptoms reveal deeper layers: a dysregulated nervous system and a body stuck in a chronic state of stress that over time has depleted your hormones and your mental bandwidth. Women are statistically twice as likely as men to experience mental health challenges like anxiety and depression, particularly during times of hormonal turbulence. Men do not have to deal with all the changing hormones throughout the month or see drastic drops in midlife like women do. As highlighted in a study published by Cambridge University Press: "Perimenopausal hormone fluctuations lead to an idiosyncratic array of physical and psychological symptoms, which may lead to new-onset mental disorders as well as affecting pre-existing conditions." Knowing that women face hormonal changes throughout their lives, we cannot afford to ignore the undeniable connection between your hormones and your overall well-being and mental health. Yet, in everyday conversations, when you ask a woman how she's doing, the default response is often, "I'm fine." But the stories I hear every day tell me otherwise.

We are not fine.

We have spent way too much time getting conditioned by the world around us on how to look, behave, move, and speak that we have lost a sense of self and have normalized feeling fine when we could feel amazing! I see women when they finally realize they can no longer function as they have been and are finally seeking the help they need, ready to drop the masks, understand their bodies, and take back their power. I hear the stories of all their discomforts, I feel the pain they have carried and the suffering they have endured, because I, too, am that woman trying to hold it all together while juggling the roles of this life; I ,too, feel the unraveling and the overwhelm of knowing I am and have been living for others while continuously abandoning myself; I, too, have ignored the signs my body was giving me for years until I couldn't ignore them any longer.

In all the unique stories that different women from different backgrounds and different circumstances experience, there are similar threads and patterns, similar expectations and similar beliefs that lead to decisions, habits, self-talk, and avoidance that have brought women from all walks of life to sit across from me to finally acknowledge that they, too, are worthy of being taken care of and need support to find themselves—or what I like to reframe it as: to remember themselves again. There are so many navigating the same waters silently and unsupported and scared to even ask for the help they deserve. Maybe out of fear, maybe out of habit, or maybe because they were rewarded for staying quiet and compliant as a child. Whatever the reason, whatever the belief that holds her back from speaking her truth, at the end of the day, this silence ends up imploding in her body and in her mind, leaving her feeling betrayed by the one person that needs to be there for her the most: HER. Your story is important, you are important.

## The Power of HER Cycle

When faced with uncomfortable symptoms, the first instinct is often to search outside ourselves for a quick fix to make the discomfort disappear. My hope is that throughout this book, you start to see how much wisdom you carry inside of you, and the answers you seek are already there. You will learn about the wisdom of your hormones and their unique rhythm in each phase of your life—the Curiosity Phase, the Vitality Phase, the Wise Woman Phase—and their rhythm in the four phases within the month—the Wisdom Keeper, the She-Warrior, the Creator, and the Nurturer—each representing an aspect of your hormones and how they support your physical and emotional well-being.

You will learn how your stories, beliefs, and your actions influence the health of your hormones, emotions, and relations. The stories you carry from the past, your own and ancestral, have a way of imprinting themselves into the present day and the lens you wear to see and experience the world around you. This perspective lens informs your beliefs, and the beliefs inform your actions through the intelligence and communication of your hormones and emotions.

This interplay is what I call the HER Cycle, a cycle that connects how those stories impact your hormones, emotions, and relations. A cycle that reminds us that your mental health is directly impacted by your hormonal health. When this cycle is disrupted by stress—whether from past trauma, societal expectations, or modern-day pressures—it can leave you feeling overwhelmed and disconnected. Stress, in all its forms—emotional, physical, or chemical—triggers your body's fight, flight, freeze, and please response.

Over time, this constant state of vigilance disrupts the delicate communication between your brain, hormones, and cells, prioritizing immediate safety over long-term healing and balance. This need for safety in your brain is amplified when your hormones are changing throughout the month and in the different phases of life, like that week before your period when everything feels overwhelming or in the throes of perimenopause. The anxiety, the depression, and the rage you may experience are a result of this cycle. This cycle changes how you show up in life—with yourself and others.

The story of stress you hold and have experienced feeds your hormones information on how to behave and how to communicate, those hormones then inform your emotions, and those emotions then influence how you experience your relations. My job as a physician has always been to find the why behind a woman's symptoms, and every single time, the investigation has led me to see how important it is to identify these stressors to break the cycle and create new circuits and new degrees of communication.

## Under Pressure: How Stress Disrupts Your Hormones

To understand the why behind how you feel, we first must understand what influences our health the most: stress. Let's take a minute to dive into how stress works so you can have this base knowledge as you continue to learn about your hormonal health in the coming chapters. Most women wake up already in a state of worry, with an endless list of tasks and the weight of perfectionism pressing down before the day even begins. This constant state of busyness and self-imposed expectations doesn't just exhaust the mind—it teaches the body to stay on high alert, fueling chronic stress and disrupting hormonal communication. Stress, whether emotional, physical, or chemical, sends a clear message through the hypothalamic-pituitary-adrenal (HPA) axis: *Survival is priority, thriving can wait.*

This constant need to keep up—powered by busyness and the endless chase for perfection—teaches your body to stay on high alert, leaving little room for rest or recovery. It may feel like a superpower that drives your productivity and keeps you going, but beneath the surface, it's quietly working against you. As you rush through your day, stress doesn't just live in your mind; it sets off a cascade of signals in your body, a deeply ingrained biological

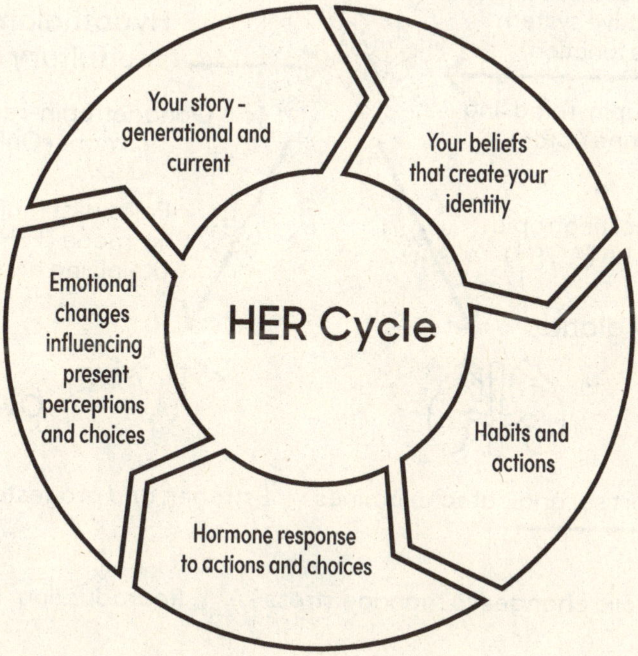

response initially designed to help you survive but now hijacked by the pace of modern life. Let's explore what happens within this system—your body's intricate stress command center—and why it often leaves you feeling exhausted, overwhelmed, and disconnected.

The HPA axis functions as your body's stress-response command center. When stress is perceived—whether it's rushing through a to-do list or feeling emotionally triggered—it activates a chain of communication between the hypothalamus, pituitary gland, and adrenal glands. This system ensures your body can respond swiftly to challenges.

Here's how it works: The amygdala, the brain's fear and emotion center, sends an alert to the hypothalamus, which releases a signal called corticotropin-releasing hormone (CRH). This signal travels to the pituitary gland, which produces adrenocorticotropic hormone (ACTH). ACTH then prompts the adrenal glands to release stress hormones like adrenaline for immediate action or cortisol for managing longer-term stress.

These hormones prepare your body to deal with perceived threats by increasing heart rate, sharpening focus, and directing energy to your muscles. However, in the process, systems like digestion, reproduction, and healing are temporarily put on hold,

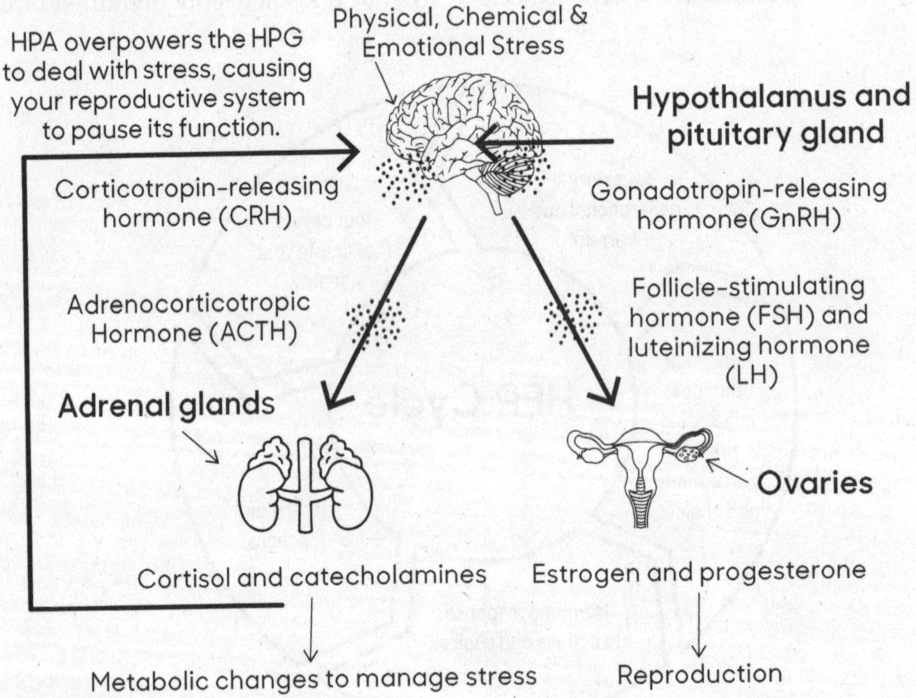

as they are considered less critical during stress. Over time, if this stress-response loop is activated too often, it can leave you feeling depleted, foggy, or out of balance. Recognizing and addressing stress is key to bringing this system back into harmony.

In small, manageable doses, stress is like lifting weights at the gym. When you pick up a heavy weight, you're intentionally creating tiny tears in your muscle fibers. This controlled stress signals your body to repair and strengthen those muscles so they're better prepared the next time you face the same challenge. This is how growth and resilience are built. Similarly, acute stress from a challenging situation—like meeting a deadline or navigating a tough conversation—can sharpen your focus and increase your ability to adapt.

But imagine lifting those weights repeatedly without rest. Instead of getting stronger, your muscles become overworked, strained, and eventually injured. Chronic stress has the same effect on your body's stress system. When your HPA axis is constantly activated, it floods your body with cortisol, the hormone designed to help you handle temporary challenges. Over time, this nonstop demand wears out your system, much like overtraining at the gym without recovery breaks. The results? Your body starts to break down—physically, emotionally, and hormonally.

Chronic stress doesn't just strain your hormonal balance; it disrupts vital systems that keep you healthy. Just like exhausted muscles lose their ability to function optimally, an overworked stress response leads to symptoms like fatigue, digestive issues, irritability, brain fog, and even lowered libido. The very system designed to protect you from harm begins to falter, leaving you feeling trapped in a cycle of "doing" without ever recharging. To truly thrive, you need to approach stress like muscle training: Challenge yourself, yes, but always allow time for recovery and healing.

Hormones are much more than just regulators of your body—they are also powerful amplifiers of your emotional experiences. When chronic stress takes hold, it doesn't just signal your body to react; it teaches your body to shut down the very processes that foster creativity, connection, and healing. This makes stress not just a temporary state but a long-term survival mode. Over time, the communication between your body and mind breaks down, much like a relationship that has been strained by demands and lacks understanding.

To truly break the cycle, it's vital to start listening to your body and honoring the signals it gives you. Giving yourself permission to rest, to heal, and to create space for thriving is key. Your hormones aren't the enemy—they're messengers trying to guide you back to balance. They're asking you to move beyond the pressure of perfection and the cycle of constant busyness, into a state where thriving is not just a goal to chase but your natural state of being. In this space, rest and rejuvenation are not weaknesses but essential components of your strength.

But to truly honor what your body is asking for, you also need to question what you've been taught to believe. By viewing your life through the lens of curiosity, you open yourself up to questioning everything you've accepted as true and the cycles that have been driving your decisions, allowing space to release what's not supporting your well-being and make room for what will. This process is what I like to call "unshoulding." You know those "shoulds"—the ones that pile up and drain you. "I should pursue this career, go to that event, eat this to look a certain way, or be this kind of mom." The pressure of these endless "shoulds" builds up over time, creating stress that impacts your hormones and feeds resentment, not just in your mind and heart but in your physical body as well.

In the upcoming chapters, you'll learn how these false identities and environmental stressors impact your emotions and organs, making it harder for your body to thrive. You'll begin to connect the dots between your past and your present, unlocking the path to your future. By the time you reach the HER Method, you'll have the tools and knowledge to commit to your healing journey, finding the freedom and balance you've been craving—mentally, emotionally, and physically.

CHAPTER 2

# The Hormonal Baggage We Inherit

Do you ever feel like you're always on high alert, ready to fight, flee, freeze, or please—even when everything seems fine? It's as if a quiet storm is brewing, and your body and mind are braced for impact. Your thoughts race, your body feels exhausted trying to keep up, and your hormones amplify every signal of alarm. For me, this heightened state has become my constant companion, especially since entering perimenopause.

What once felt like occasional stress now defines my daily life, shaping how I see myself and interact with those around me. Impatience, a persistent sense of dread, waves of grief, and a loss of control have become all too familiar. It's reminiscent of the turmoil of puberty—a time when your body and emotions seemed to take over, leaving you powerless to stop the changes.

As someone who has lived through trauma, I've come to recognize how deeply my responses today are rooted in the body's protective mechanisms just as we learned in the previous chapter about the function of stress. These feelings often resurface when I don't feel safe in my environment or within myself. But what I didn't fully grasp until years into my healing journey is how intimately these patterns are tied to the lives of the women who came before me. The struggles they endured, the traumas they faced, and the survival strategies they used have been passed down through generations, embedding themselves in my cells and shaping my emotional and physical landscape.

**The trauma of the mother becomes the trauma of the daughter**, whether it's consciously passed down or inherited through generations of unresolved pain. Some of the behaviors may be from mirroring reactions we have seen while others are from the biological connection from grandmother to daughter and to granddaughter—through the hormonal dialogue between the generations and women's bodies. Understanding this dynamic is key to breaking the cycle and healing.

When we trace the emotional and physical patterns we experience back to our mothers and grandmothers, we realize that their struggles—whether related to stress, survival, societal expectations, or emotional turmoil—don't just affect them. They *live* inside us, shaping how we interact with our own world. How they navigated stress and their reaction to it become our own unconscious reactions. If you witnessed that stress was best dealt with through irritation, or passive-aggressive behavior like silent treatments or angry outbursts, if you pause and reflect on your own responses today, you may notice some similarities. Understanding that what you are feeling today may not only be rooted in your own life experiences but also in the inherited stories of your lineage opens the door to deep healing and understanding of yourself.

As you begin to connect with your ancestors' wounds, you begin to rewrite the patterns that no longer serve you and take steps toward releasing the stories you no longer need to carry. The unhealed trauma and patterns of one generation often become the hidden inheritance of the next. If your mother struggled with anxiety, or if she had to endure emotional pain without tools to process it, you might find yourself carrying the weight of those unresolved emotions. This process of generational trauma creates a powerful link between mother and daughter, one that has profound effects on our physical, emotional, and mental health.

Take Rachel's story, for example. On the outside, she seems to have it all—successful career, family, a lovely home—but inside, she feels anxious and hopeless. She has had struggles with infertility, multiple miscarriages, and now perimenopausal symptoms like extreme fatigue and low libido. Despite managing her family and career, she hit a wall. As we started to work together, she realized her constant need to be perfect and busy came from a deep-seated fear of not being enough—a fear that stemmed from her childhood. Her mother, who also dealt with stress and modeled perfectionism, had her own health problems and had passed down these patterns and expectations. Rachel's healing began when she recognized that the stress and patterns she inherited from her mother weren't hers to carry anymore.

By looking at her family history and understanding these inherited patterns, over time she was able to release the burden of perfectionism. She learned to pause before reacting with her usual pattern of saying yes to everything and learned to question her own beliefs. The moment she realized that she didn't have to repeat the cycles of stress from her past, she was able to make room for self-care, self-awareness, and self-acceptance. She started to believe that she could make daily choices to support her mental and physical health without feeling guilty, and she learned to say no. No to anything that was depleting her and making room for what was nurturing her—healing foods, movement, and uplifting relationships—and, most importantly, she learned to ask for help—a vulnerability that was never accepted in her childhood home.

This chapter will explore how the trauma of our mothers and the women before them becomes our own, and how understanding and healing these patterns can lead to a life of peace and empowerment, free from the chains of inherited suffering. The stories of the women who came before us are embedded in our bodies, and by acknowledging them, we can find the wisdom to break the cycle and transform our health, relationships, and futures.

## The Generational Thread

I once heard a story about lovers and what happens when the communication between them breaks down and they begin to yell at each other in anger. Sufi teaching says that the reason why we shout even though we are right next to another and are physically close is that the hearts have become so far apart, and we have created so much space between them that we must yell to make up the distance. On the other side, when we are in a loving relationship and our heart is very close to someone, we can be in the same room and not have to say a word, and the other knows exactly what is on your mind. When two hearts are close, there's no desire to yell, but just a whisper helps you feel safe, heard, and seen. This is also the story of your cells and your hormones. The clearer the communication from healthy habits, stress management, and generational healing, the healthier the cells and the healthier the hormones.

Hormones, as messengers within the body, respond not just to the immediate environment but also to deeper, more ingrained factors—including the generational stories and beliefs passed down through families. These inherited stories, shaped by past experiences, cultural conditioning, and societal expectations, become imprinted in your cells over time. This can create a subtle yet powerful influence on your biology.

Just as your hormones communicate with the cells to orchestrate bodily functions, these generational stories impact how your cells respond to stress and health. We inherit more than just physical traits; we inherit the emotional and psychological patterns of those who came before us. These inherited patterns can influence how we process stress, how we respond to challenges, and even how we experience health issues.

For example, if a family has a long history of women who were taught to "push through" or suppress emotions, this belief becomes encoded not just in the mind but in the very cells that respond to stress. This might manifest in chronic stress, hormonal imbalances, or emotional depletion, as the body's systems react to the story of perpetual striving, neglecting rest, or the avoidance of vulnerability.

The hormones, ever sensitive to the environment they're placed in, will reflect these generational beliefs, either nurturing or disrupting the body's balance. When the environment is one of unresolved trauma or limiting beliefs, the hormones "yell" in response, signaling distress through physical and emotional symptoms like anxiety, weight changes, and digestive issues. These stressors, deeply rooted in family history, echo through the body and influence how it manages stress, signaling the need for healing and transformation.

Thus, generational stories become part of the internal environment in which your hormones function, influencing how your cells "listen" to the messages and how they respond. Healing the body requires not only tending to the physical environment but also understanding and releasing the inherited stories and beliefs that may have been passed down for generations.

Generational threads are the stories and behaviors we inherit, and these invisible threads tether us to the past, influencing our sense of safety, belonging, and self-worth in ways we often don't consciously understand. For example, if your lineage carries a story of needing to work tirelessly to be valued, you might find yourself locked into cycles of overworking and overgiving, driven by an inherited sense of duty or fear of not being enough. This inherited stress can leave traces on your hormonal health, keeping you stuck in a fight-or-flight system—manifesting as thyroid imbalances, menstrual issues, or chronic fatigue—patterns often mirrored across generations.

Healing the HER Cycle requires breaking these generational patterns. It begins with curiosity and compassion—learning to see the connection between the way your body reacts to stress and the stories that shaped your family's identity. By recognizing these narratives, you can consciously choose which to release and which to transform. This work is not only for you but for the generations that follow, allowing them to inherit a new story—one of balance, health, and self-worth.

A story of a patient comes to mind that describes this thread perfectly. Stella, 87 years old, presented a long list of health concerns: high blood pressure, anxiety, constipation, and more. When asked about her past, she opened up about a life shaped by profound resilience and sacrifice. She shared her journey of immigration, leaving everything familiar behind to build a life for her family from scratch. She recounted moments of extreme danger, including having a gun pointed at her during war, and dreams she willingly set aside for her children.

This rich tapestry of her life revealed not just struggles but also profound strength. As she spoke, it became clear how her body carried the imprints of these experiences, echoing unprocessed stress and sacrifice through her health symptoms. Her story wasn't just hers—it was also woven into the lives of her daughter and granddaughter. Her daughter, overwhelmed by the dual roles of caretaker and career woman, juggled the inherited pressures of overachieving and self-sacrifice, while her granddaughter grappled with similar emotional and physical patterns, such as menstrual and thyroid challenges.

Stella's story also highlights the silent transmission of generational narratives. For her, the sacrifices she made became a form of love; for her daughter, they became a template for survival. However, survival often came at the expense of emotional and physical well-being, showing up in their shared health issues and stress responses.

When hearing Stella's stories—her strength, joys, and challenges—her daughter began to see her not just as a mother but as a whole woman. This shift in perspective helped untangle the emotional threads of obligation and guilt and offered space for compassion and healing. It also opened the door to breaking cycles of overwork, emotional suppression, and inherited stress, allowing new patterns of health, balance, and self-awareness to emerge.

This is the essence of addressing generational threads: recognizing that while these stories shape us, they don't have to define us. By consciously choosing to understand and rewrite these narratives, we not only heal our own HER Cycles but also gift future generations with the freedom to live healthier and more aligned lives.

## Changing the Inherited Story

It's remarkable how storytelling is woven into the fabric of cultures across time. In the past, stories shared by elders around fires were threads that bound communities, passing down wisdom and shaping identities. Today, storytelling often looks different. Instead of gathering in circles, we absorb narratives from the glowing screens in our hands. These modern stories—whether from influencers, advertisements, or fleeting social media posts—are now shaping how we perceive ourselves, our health, and our relationships.

The power of storytelling lies in its ability to inform how we see our worth, our place in society, and our choices. But here's the challenge: If the storytellers of previous generations or today's digital age haven't done the work to reflect on and heal their own inherited patterns, we inherit their unresolved narratives. These can create limiting beliefs that resonate through our cells, influencing everything from how we navigate stress to how we nurture relationships. This becomes the generational thread: the invisible but tangible connection between past stories and present-day experiences.

Generational stories, particularly those rooted in trauma, can have a profound impact on our health and ability to heal. Research into intergenerational trauma has shown how the stress endured by one generation can influence the biology of the next, particularly in how the body manages stress hormones. This connection between past experiences and present-day health highlights how deeply we carry the emotional and physical legacies of those who came before us. Later in this chapter, I'll delve deeper into the work of experts like Rachel Yehuda, whose research illuminates how trauma reshapes biology across generations. For now, consider this: If the struggles and survival mechanisms of our ancestors can influence our stress responses, could their resilience and strength also hold keys to healing? By reflecting on our own HER-stories and those of the women who came before us, we may uncover not just the burdens but also the wisdom necessary to write a new narrative for ourselves.

To change the cycle and rewrite your story, it's essential to pause and examine the beliefs we've inherited. What were the stories whispered by your ancestors? Were they empowering, or were they shaped by survival, sacrifice, and fear? By quieting external noise from old narratives, we can tune in to our own inner wisdom. This allows us to break free from patterns that have kept us disconnected and stuck in a cycle of stress and reaction. This story that you are rewriting weaves together the history of your lineage with the present-day experiences that influence your health and well-being. It reveals how the generational narratives of our ancestors—their struggles, triumphs, and adaptations—are embedded in our biology and inform our health today, especially our hormonal health.

These ancestral experiences are carried in our cells, shaping the way our bodies react to stress and regulate hormones. For example, the history of famine among South Asians led to genetic changes that now affect beta-cell function in the pancreas, possibly contributing to higher rates of insulin resistance and diabetes—making them susceptible to heart disease and other conditions. This biological adaptation was a response to survival but now poses challenges in modern lifestyles, especially during hormonal transitions like perimenopause, when the body is losing its hormonal armor, leaving it vulnerable to express hidden stories of *dis-ease.*

Every lineage has its HERstory that informs who we are today. Honoring these stories helps us understand ourselves and our health better. By reflecting on the past, we gain insight into patterns, uncover strengths, and learn how to break cycles that no longer serve us.

Understanding your lineage helps you see the bigger picture: the strengths passed down, the adaptations that supported survival, and the choices you can now make to rewrite your narrative for yourself and future generations. It's about embracing your history, not as a burden but as a source of wisdom and empowerment.

## Womb Wisdom

Your first direct environment of influence is your mother's womb. Her state—mental, emotional, and physical—impacts that environment through hormonal changes, immune cells, nutrients, and even toxins. The placenta, the interface between the mother and fetus, is one of the most important organs of the body and is the place of connection between the maternal and fetal blood flow. It acts as detoxifier, a nutrient metabolizer, and an oxygen-exchange site to keep the fetus healthy and thriving and is a major endocrine organ that not only receives signals from the maternal blood but gives out signals through various hormones. If you have been pregnant or know someone that has, you've heard or experienced some of the common stories. (I don't like calling them symptoms, as pregnancy isn't a disease—it is a major superpower!) These include increased appetite, more fat deposition, fatigue, aches and pains, nausea (there are some lucky ones who get to skip this), and mostly a feeling of not being in control of one's body and even choices (children start calling the shots right from the beginning!).

These changes are orchestrated by that hormonal dance and by the input of a mother's current and historical environment. The input that you received didn't start in your mother's womb, but in your grandmother's. When she was pregnant with your mother, you were already being created in your mother's ovaries—how wild is that! So that connection between you and your maternal grandmother starts sooner than you think, and her health and her choices and experiences started shaping your story then.

This matrilineal thread—where biology, experience, and energy are passed down—exists not just in our bodies, but in the rhythms that surround us. And no rhythm has guided women more intimately than that of Grandmother Moon—a title of reverence given to the moon by Native peoples. Having studied the shamanic medicine wheel, I have come to understand how these cultures so beautifully see all things and all relations as connected. They see the spirit in all and have connected the moon to women because of its power over the waters of the earth. Just as birth happens through water—as it is the first environment we live in and that influences our growth—so, too, does the moon shift the tides of this earth and all things living on it. The moon governs the seasons; she tells us when it is time to harvest and when it is time to seed. She connects us to the cycles of the earth, just as she connects women to the cycles of their bleed.

The moon is a guide through the darkness and has gifted women with the wisdom of her cycle. This topic remains controversial in the world of science but is understood deeply in the world of spirit. Long-term studies have been done to explore the connection between the moon's phases and menstrual cycle onset. What's become clear is that, in ancient times, when women lived more closely aligned with the rhythms of the natural world, this synchronicity was stronger. In contrast, modern living—with artificial light, stress, and overstimulation—has dulled that connection for many.

When studying a woman's cycle, many factors can influence its length and timing: from what she eats, to where she travels, to the level of stress she carries, and even her bedtime routine. These internal and external influences can pull us out of rhythm—with the moon, and with our bodies. Yet the wisdom remains. The connection to Grandmother Moon remains. It lives within us. And through daily choices, we either drift farther from it—or come closer.

This connection to rhythm, to water, to cycles—it all begins before we even take our first breath. A woman's first experience of life is inside her mother's womb, suspended in water, held by rhythm, shaped by sound and sensation. Before she ever bleeds with the moon, she is already receiving its wisdom through the tides of her mother's body. Regardless of your relationship with your mother today, her body once made space for you to swim in its waters. Her heartbeat gave you rhythm—a drumbeat that called your soul into form and reminded you of home. That was your first environment of influence. And that wisdom is still inside you.

As we move through this book together, my hope is that you find ways to reconnect to that inner wisdom—to remember what your body has always known and return home to the rhythms that are yours by birthright.

## What She Carried, You Became

The environment you developed in—the womb—was already shaped by layers of influence: your mother's mindset, her emotional health, her nutrition, and even her relationship with her own mother. These early influences, along with inherited trauma, environmental toxins, and cultural stressors, helped shape the hormonal patterns and cellular environment that would become yours.

The above influences, as we know now through the work of Bruce Lipton and epigenetics, work on changing the environment of your cells. These changes occur according to the daily choices that will either create an environment where your cells can thrive and keep the "bad" genes that can lead to ailments like cancer quiet or create an environment where these "bad" genes can thrive, creating chaos in the body. What you may not be aware of is that the actions, thoughts, and circumstances and the choices of your parents and grandparents can have influence over how your hormones communicate and function, impacting the environment of those genes. Some choices and life circumstances will create resilience and strength in this system, while others will create changes that deplete it.

Trauma, including generational trauma, plays a significant but often overlooked role in hormonal health. Rachel Yehuda, a leading researcher in psychiatry and neuroscience, has studied how trauma from one generation can influence the hormonal systems of the next. Her work highlights the impact on the hypothalamic-pituitary-adrenal (HPA) axis, the body's central stress-response system, which is programmed

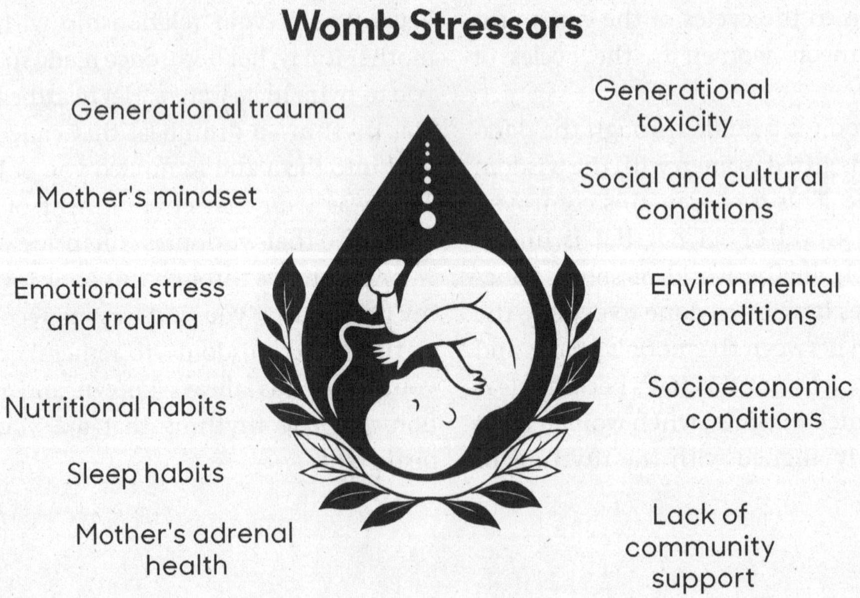

during fetal development and can shape long-term health outcomes.

When a mother experiences heightened stress, her adrenal glands release elevated levels of glucocorticoids, such as cortisol. These stress hormones can affect the developing HPA axis of the fetus, increasing the child's risk of future issues like metabolic syndrome, high blood pressure, glucose intolerance, and imbalanced lipid levels. Research into children of Holocaust survivors, for example, reveals a pattern of low cortisol levels paired with heightened glucocorticoid receptor sensitivity. This adaptation, likely a response to the trauma, alters how these individuals handle stress, impacts their neuronal circuitry, and creates a predisposition to mood disorders like anxiety and depression. It also disrupts sex hormone regulation, contributing to symptoms such as heavy periods, insomnia, and low libido.

Importantly, trauma doesn't have to stem from major life events. Studies show that mothers' experiences of childhood microtraumas and emotional abuse can lead to heightened sympathetic nervous system activation in their offspring, predisposing them to anxiety and stress-related vulnerabilities. This underscores how a mother's environment and stress levels can profoundly influence her child's health. In one study, researchers looked at the cortisol-awakening response (CAR) score of pregnant mothers—the rapid increase in cortisol within 30 minutes of being awake. Researchers then tested the CAR scores of their infants all the way up to nine months of age to see if there were any correlations between their scores with their mothers'. What was found was that infants born to mothers with low CAR scores had a more difficult time adapting to stress, the low scores reflected a state of chronic stress in the mother that translated into altered behavior in the infant. This finding shows the direct correlation between a mother's stress levels and her child's capacity to manage and cope with stress as they develop.

When we think about intergenerational trauma, we might picture major historical events like colonization, wars, or famines. But trauma can also stem from everyday challenges. Situations where a child feels unsafe, unseen, or afraid leave lasting imprints on their biology, shaping how they adapt to stress in the future. This is the body's way of ensuring survival by preparing for similar challenges. For instance, a child growing up in a home with an alcoholic parent, a caregiver overwhelmed by stress, or one working multiple jobs to make ends meet may develop adaptive behaviors to navigate these dynamics. They might learn to suppress their own needs, avoid conflict, or strive for peace at all costs. These patterns are rooted in the brain's response to stress, activating the sympathetic nervous system (the fight-or-flight mode) and leaving less space for the development of trust and safety circuits. This ongoing stress can also disrupt the balance and development of their hormones, influencing emotional and physical health as they grow.

We've explored ancestral stories, early life influences, and even the impact of the womb—now it's time to examine how everyday experiences shape us. From a young age, children mirror the behaviors, emotions, and habits of those around them, creating deep neural connections through specialized brain cells called *mirror neurons*. These neurons allow us to emotionally sync with others, like tearing up when a loved one cries or feeling anger in a crowd protesting for a cause. Mirror neurons develop early, before a child turns one, and continue shaping their understanding of the world as they grow, helping them learn social norms and behaviors by observing parents, teachers, and other influential people in their lives.

What we hear and see—especially stories and responses to stress—deeply influences how we think, feel, and act. Research shows that listening to the same story can synchronize brain activity across individuals, highlighting the power of the voices and stories we allow into our lives. Amplifying the voice of the narrator. These mirror neurons wire together, shaping our perception and driving our habits, behaviors, and ultimately our biology. From how we eat and move to how we handle emotions, these patterns influence our hormones and their ability to communicate and define how we show up each day.

CHAPTER 3

# "Women Are Just Too Emotional . . ."

"I'm done fighting my depression." These were the first words Kelly, a 42-year-old woman, said to me, her voice breaking as she fought back her tears. For years, she had tried everything—different medications, therapies, and strategies—but nothing seemed to free her from the dark cloud that loomed over her life. Despite her efforts, the depression lingered, stealing her ability to be present, straining her relationships, and leaving her feeling powerless. Every day felt like a battle she was losing, and the sense of defeat was magnified in the week before her period. During those days, her world turned colorless, and she felt overwhelmed by a wave of self-doubt and comparison, convinced that everyone around her had it together while she crumbled.

Yet, she noticed something remarkable. As soon as her period began, it was as if the fog lifted—she could feel glimpses of joy and connection again. That realization gave her a spark of hope, one that brought her to me, ready to explore the deeper connection between her emotional state, her cycle, and her hormones. She wanted to understand why she felt the way she did and reclaim her life.

Hope became Kelly's anchor. It wasn't about finding a quick fix but about creating a new relationship with her depression—one rooted in curiosity, compassion, and small, intentional steps forward. By supporting her body with nutrient-dense foods that balanced her hormones, exercising to boost endorphins, and incorporating bioidentical hormones and supplements, she started to notice shifts. Days of clarity and energy became more frequent, helping her rebuild trust in herself and her ability to navigate life's challenges.

Through this process, Kelly realized that hope isn't an illusion but a powerful tool—a way to transform despair into strength and presence. It helped her shift from a place of suffering to one of empowerment, showing her that even in her darkest moments, she could make choices to stand in her power.

Could understanding your emotions and learning to work with them be the antidote to physical, emotional, and mental suffering? Over years of working with women and children, it's clear that how we manage our emotional state shapes our health, relationships, and life. Suffering from those emotions often emerges when we fail to see the wisdom within our challenges.

As humans, we are wired to avoid pain and pursue pleasure. But in this pursuit, we often mold ourselves to fit in, adapting to what's expected to avoid the pain of rejection or not belonging. From a young age, we learn to suppress our needs or desires if they create conflict, often silencing our voices to maintain harmony. This survival mechanism—hiding our truth to belong—carries into adulthood, influencing how we navigate our relationships, work, and even our health. For many women, this pattern of silencing their voices shows up starkly in the doctor's office. The fear of being dismissed, labeled as "too emotional," or told "it's all in your head" causes them to downplay their symptoms or refrain from fully expressing how they're feeling. This need to appease and avoid confrontation mirrors societal conditioning that teaches women to prioritize others' comfort over their own needs. As a result, women often leave appointments feeling unheard, misunderstood, or powerless.

True healing requires us to break this cycle—to confront the fear of not belonging among others and reclaim our voice. This journey is not easy, but it is necessary. Bravery in this context means asking questions even when it feels uncomfortable, expressing your needs even when they seem "too much," and advocating for your health even when met with resistance, and most importantly, befriending those uncomfortable emotions you have tried so hard to avoid. Hope really is the bridge that carries us forward. It is the nectar we must drink daily, allowing us to rebuild trust in ourselves, our intuition, and the emotions that guide us. In that trust, we find the courage to be seen and heard, opening the door to transformation and healing.

## Tearing Off the Mask

Do you ever look at others and wonder, *Why can't I have it all together like they do?* When we compare instead of connect, we lose sight of our own strengths and gifts, yearning to mold ourselves into someone else's version of success. This longing often comes from a deep need to belong, to avoid the pain of rejection or isolation. It's a survival instinct—if we fit in, we stay safe. But this safety comes at a cost: We end up wearing masks to please others, conform, and hide our true selves.

So many of us walk through life projecting happiness and perfection while suppressing our pain, discomfort, and desires. In this act of masking, we forget the truth: Beneath it all, we share the same fundamental needs—to be loved, supported, heard, and to belong. These universal needs are expressed through our emotions, the common language of the human soul. Whether it's joy, grief, anger, or love, emotions are what connect us as humans. They can unite us or tear us apart, but they are always calling us to listen and come home to ourselves.

I often see women struggling with their emotions, feeling completely out of control—especially during specific phases of their cycles or pivotal stages of life. It can feel like you're being momentarily hijacked—when you snap at a partner for chewing loudly, lose patience with a toddler, or feel defeated by pants that no longer fit. Even though there's a voice inside urging you to pause and reflect, the emotional hijacker often wins, leaving you with regret and disappointment in yourself.

But what if we approached these moments differently? What if that anger, frustration, or sadness is your body's way of sending you a message? Perhaps there are unresolved feelings you've been ignoring, overwhelming responsibilities piling up, or truths you've been too afraid to voice. By pausing and asking our emotions questions, we can use them as tools for growth and healing.

The real challenge is that we haven't been taught to understand our emotions, and most of what we know comes from the environments we grew up in. But emotions, much like a teeter-totter, shift and sway, allowing us to experience the full spectrum of life. In striving for perfection and avoiding discomfort, we silence the very emotions that are trying to wake us up and guide us toward possibility.

What if we started seeing emotions as allies instead of enemies? Imagine if, from a young age, we were taught to embrace them as teachers. By exploring their role in our mental, physical, and relational health, we could build emotional resilience. This wisdom would ripple through every decision we make, every relationship we nurture, and every aspect of life. It's in this shift—from merely surviving to thriving—that we uncover the freedom to live as our truest selves.

## What Is an Emotion?

How would you define an emotion? Is it a state, a reaction, a perception, a fleeting electric signal in the brain, or a condition deeply tied to our human experience? From a young age, we are taught to recognize emotions by using simple tools like the little round faces on posters in classrooms. These early lessons often reduce emotions to basic categories: happy, sad, or mad, leaving much of their complexity unexplored.

As we grow, we begin to experience emotions in layers, their power shaping how we interact with the world. Life moves from the simplicity of black and white into a spectrum of vivid colors as we encounter more nuanced emotional states. By reflecting on the emotions we sit in most often or the ones we default to when navigating challenges, we can start to uncover deeper truths about our stories and our inner worlds. Understanding this connection can reveal patterns—how certain emotions dominate our responses and why they hold that power. It's like finding out who's directing your internal narrative and opening a door to self-awareness and growth.

For example, let's take the emotion of sadness. When you hear the word, it might immediately evoke a memory, a feeling, or the image of someone experiencing it. We often associate sadness with loss, disappointment, or negativity—a state where we feel "down." But what if we redefined sadness?

John Koenig's *The Dictionary of Obscure Sorrows* offers a different perspective. The word *sadness* originally meant "fullness," stemming from the Latin root *satis*, which also gives us the word *satisfaction*. Sadness, in its essence, was about being so filled with emotion that joy and grief could coexist in one experience or moment. Think about it: The sadness you feel after an argument with your partner could also remind you of the joy and connection you share. The sadness when your kids leave home reflects the fullness of those cherished moments. Or the sadness after a loss—it's a testament to the love and significance of what was. This shift in perception allows sadness to become more than a heavy feeling; it becomes a reminder of connection, meaning, and possibility. The next time you feel sad after a disagreement or a challenging experience, pause and ask yourself: *What am I really longing for? What do I feel is lost, and what could I reclaim?* Often, the answer lies in a desire for connection—whether with yourself or others.

Emotions like sadness, anxiety, or grief—and even joy, gratitude, and peace—are not just fleeting states. They're messengers. They speak to what matters, reflect our intuition, and guide us toward self-awareness. By understanding these emotions, we deepen our relationship with ourselves, using them as tools to navigate life's ups and downs with more intention and clarity.

Emotions aren't just felt in the mind—they are created through a delicate balance of **hormones** and **neurotransmitters**, the body's chemical messengers. This internal chemistry influences everything from your mood and energy to how your body handles stress. When this balance is disrupted, it can lead to emotional highs and lows, anxiety, fatigue, and even physical symptoms.

Scientist and physician Esther Sternberg has spent years studying this connection, showing how closely our emotional experiences are tied to the chemical signals in our brain and body. Understanding these biochemical messengers allows us to grasp how they shape our perceptions and experiences. Neurotransmitters are chemical signals used by the nervous system to facilitate communication between nerve cells. When one nerve releases a neurotransmitter, it signals the next nerve, which triggers a response in the body. For instance, serotonin is a neurotransmitter that plays a role in mood regulation, sleep, digestion, and even cardiovascular health. When released, serotonin can influence gut motility and promote a sense of relaxation or happiness. Medications like selective serotonin reuptake inhibitors (SSRIs), commonly prescribed for depression, especially for women, work by prolonging the presence of serotonin in the brain's communication channels, the synaptic clefts. This mechanism helps sustain feelings of happiness and reduces the prevalence of sadness. When your hormones fluctuate, so do your neurotransmitters, equating to changes in your emotional state.

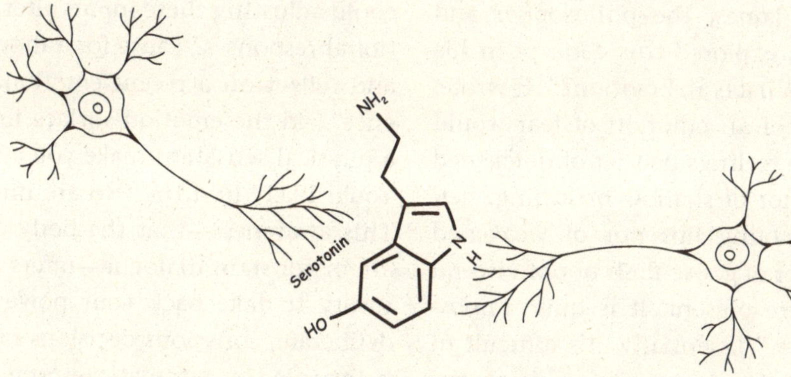


Synaptic cleft releases the neurotransmitter in need from the presynaptic cleft to the postsynaptic cleft of the next neuron.

The question to ask then is—do emotions come first, or does a physiological change signal the brain to release certain hormones and neurotransmitters, creating the emotion in response to an experience? Think about the anxiety you might feel a week before your period, the sadness following a hysterectomy, or the rage during perimenopause. Is the emotion influencing the hormones, or are the hormonal shifts eliciting emotions to signal that something needs attention?

This interplay between emotions and physiology is not one-directional; instead, it forms a dynamic feedback loop. Hormonal shifts, such as those in the luteal phase of the menstrual cycle or during perimenopause, can amplify emotional responses, making feelings like anxiety, irritability, or sadness more intense. At the same time, our emotions—shaped by life experiences, trauma, or daily stressors—can alter hormonal pathways, reinforcing patterns of stress or imbalance. Understanding this bidirectional relationship is key to recognizing how deeply our emotional and physical states are intertwined and why addressing both can be transformative for our well-being.

For instance, when you momentarily lose sight of your child in a crowded room, your heart rate spikes, your stomach churns, and a wave of panic overtakes you. These physical sensations—the racing heart, shallow breaths, and tightened chest—are triggered by a flood of stress hormones like adrenaline and cortisol. Only after these sensations register does your brain interpret them as fear and spring into action to find your child. Similarly, the trembling hands and flushed cheeks during an argument are your body's initial response, signaling the brain to process the emotions of anger or frustration. These interactions between the body and mind create a feedback loop, with each experience shaping how your brain and body respond the next time, reinforcing patterns and emotional habits.

William James, the philosopher and psychologist, explored this concept in his 1884 essay "What Is an Emotion?" He wrote: "What kind of an emotion of fear would be left, if the feelings neither of quickened heart-beats nor of shallow breathing, neither of trembling lips nor of weakened limbs, neither of goose-flesh nor of visceral stirrings, were present, it is quite impossible to think." Essentially, it's difficult to separate emotional experiences from the physical sensations and the changes that accompany them.

The body and mind are constantly engaged in this dynamic conversation, with physical sensations triggering emotions and emotional responses influencing physiological patterns. This interplay becomes particularly significant when we consider the hormonal shifts women experience throughout their lives—shifts that are often mirrored in their emotional states. Think of the grief you might feel as you notice changes in your body throughout the month or in stages like perimenopause—the hormonal weight gain, wrinkling skin, or thinning hair—or the heat rising in your chest during moments of irritability with your partner. Could these emotional reactions stem from shifting hormones? If so, what is influencing these changing hormones? Your hormones respond to environmental inputs, like the stressors we identified earlier—emotional, chemical, and physical. These include diet, exposure to toxins, or even habits like people-pleasing—all of which can shape your hormonal balance and, in turn, your emotional states. So, could adjusting these inputs alter our emotional responses? Pause for a moment here and reflect on a recent emotional experience. Did the emotion surface first, or did a physical sensation make you aware of it? You'll likely find the two are intertwined. This awareness—that the body and mind are in constant dialogue—offers an opportunity to take back your power, making deliberate, conscious decisions rather than being ruled by automatic responses.

As I reflect on this profound interplay and listen to the stories shared by my patients, it becomes increasingly clear that our emotions and physical experiences are not separate entities but deeply interconnected. A woman's attachment to her former sense of vitality—whether it's her once-thick hair, once-youthful skin, or once-strong physique—is often rooted in hormonal changes that have been subtly shaped by environmental influences. These can include toxins, trauma, and the internalized messages from thoughts and societal pressures. The emotions that arise—grief, anger, resentment—are not simply reactions; they are guiding forces. They help her assign meaning to her experiences and serve as a call to action, pushing her toward self-awareness, healing, and a deeper understanding of her authentic self.

Hormones, in their intricate dance with the mind, shape the way we perceive the world. They don't merely affect our physical state; they filter our experiences through the lens of our emotions, coloring everything we see, feel, and react to. In this way, emotions become the key to unlocking not just our personal narratives, but the potential for profound transformation and healing.

## Emotions—Your Superpower

Have you ever experienced emotions so overwhelming that they seem to consume your entire being? Perhaps it was an intense love for your child, fiery rage at an injustice, deep empathy for a struggling neighbor, or seething anger toward a partner. These emotions can feel so powerful that they leave you shaking, desperate for an outlet to transform or release them. Yet, each emotion carries its own purpose and potential. Anger can be a call to action, rage a demand for change, grief a reminder of gratitude, and worry an invitation for reflection. These feelings, when understood and harnessed, offer opportunities for growth. But when left unmanaged, they can control and even harm us.

In Ayurvedic medicine, an ancient healing tradition from India, it is believed that the inability to understand or navigate emotions is a central cause of imbalance in the body. Emotions shape how we perceive our environment and guide the decisions we make. Take, for example, the week before your period, when irritability and frustration may take center stage. These emotions not only color your interactions with your partner, children, or even yourself, but they also validate your thoughts and assumptions, creating a feedback loop between the emotional centers of your brain and your hormonal system. This loop influences how you act—whether to amplify or defuse the emotions you're experiencing.

Emotions drive so many aspects of our daily lives, which makes understanding their triggers crucial. Through my work with thousands of women, I've learned that stress—and, more importantly, how we respond to it—is a universal factor influencing both hormonal and emotional shifts. It's not just external stressors that matter, but how we internalize them and react. By acknowledging this connection, we can start to unravel the cycles that drain us and take active steps toward healing and regaining balance.

Consider the belief "I am not enough." This deeply ingrained core belief for many women often narrates our inner dialogue throughout the day, shaping how we interpret everyday challenges and contributing to our stress. For instance, when you see a pile of unwashed laundry, miss a deadline at work, forget a school project for your child, or blank on the name of a familiar mom at the playground, the default thought might be *I'm a failure,* or *Of course I'm not enough.* This thought feels validated, often triggering emotions like anger or resentment—toward yourself or your situation.

This belief-driven stress activates your body's stress-response system, known as the HPA axis, sending a signal to your brain's emotional center, the amygdala. The amygdala reinforces your habitual feelings associated with this belief, reigniting anger and solidifying the cycle. Over time, repeated activation of this system doesn't just impact your emotions—it also affects your physical health. For example, research has shown that such stress increases levels of interleukin-6 (IL-6), a pro-inflammatory cytokine linked to immune dysfunction and cardiovascular strain.

A study published in 2014 stated that women with low social support are at higher risk of increased IL-6 in response to anger. The women in the study were exposed to a trigger at different time intervals and assessed for emotions of fear, anger, and anxiety and their connection to IL-6. Only anger seemed to influence the increase in IL-6, making them vulnerable to inflammation. What was brilliant to see was that if these women received support and connection, their connection between anger and IL-6 went down. So, once again proving that connection and compassion in our relations, especially the one we have with ourselves, can be emotionally and physically healing, and that disconnection can reinforce damaging cycles.

Take Stacey's story, for instance. This woman in her 40s came to me overwhelmed by the toll her body and emotions were taking on her life. She was deep into perimenopause and experiencing incredibly heavy periods—so heavy that even the most absorbent pads couldn't prevent leaks. This wasn't just a physical challenge; it was reshaping her entire life. The bleeding would last over a week, and the buildup was filled with debilitating cramping, anxiety, and waves of depression. She felt irritable, snapping at her family and retreating from the world. Her family didn't know how to approach her, and she didn't know how to escape the constant cycle of pain and frustration. Despite this, life didn't pause for her. Work, motherhood, and relationships all demanded her energy, which was already running on empty.

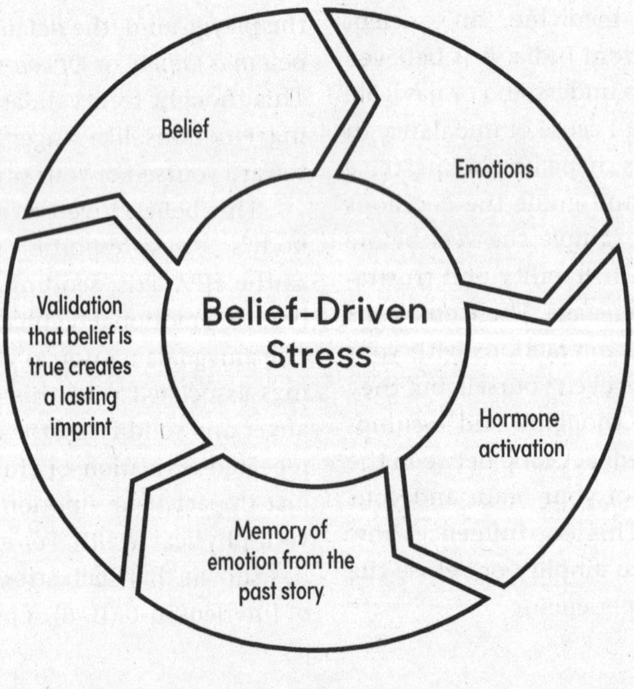

After investigating, we discovered she had large fibroids and hormonal imbalances, particularly estrogen dominance. Her estrogen wasn't breaking down properly, and her progesterone—responsible for keeping her calm and balanced—was unable to do its job. When I asked about her stress, she explained that since turning 40, she had lost her ability to keep up with her demanding life. Tasks that once felt manageable—like working long hours, chauffeuring her kids, cooking dinner, and staying social—now left her drained. She couldn't bounce back from sleepless nights, and her body seemed to have hit the brakes.

Her self-worth, tied so tightly to her ability to "do it all," crumbled. She hated herself for not meeting her own expectations. As we dug deeper, it became clear this wasn't just about her present struggles. Her childhood experiences shaped her drive for perfection. She shared how growing up, anything less than perfect brought rejection or punishment. Her stress response was rooted in those early survival mechanisms, where pleasing others became her way of avoiding pain.

I explained how trauma like hers can create a constant state of vigilance, keeping the body focused on survival. This shifts hormonal priorities—pushing stress hormones to the forefront and leaving little room for healing and balance. I also shared a study conducted by the Boston University School of Medicine, which followed 60,000 women over 16 years. The study found that women who experienced childhood trauma, such as abuse or neglect, were significantly more likely to develop uterine fibroids as adults. It demonstrated how emotional stress from childhood alters physiology, influencing hormone function and increasing inflammation. This connection between early trauma and Stacey's current health helped her understand that her heavy periods weren't just random—they were deeply tied to her life story.

Over time, stress impacts choices, from food habits to how we handle daily challenges, creating a cycle of depletion and imbalance. For Stacey, it had been years of pushing herself, relying on caffeine to power through mornings and wine to unwind at night, that contributed to her symptoms screaming for attention.

Understanding this connection helped her begin to heal. At first, she felt grief—grieving for the years lost to overwhelm, the time she had felt absent from her kids' lives, and the joy she had missed while striving to please everyone. But as she worked through her emotions, she found gratitude for her body's resilience. She realized her body had been signaling her all along, and now, with the right support, she was ready to listen.

Over several months, through physical and emotional healing and using the HER Method, a method detailed in coming chapters, she completely transformed. Her periods became manageable, her fibroids shrank, and her relationship with herself shifted. She began speaking her truth, felt closer to her partner, and became more present for her children. Most importantly, she reclaimed her worth and stepped into a life filled with gratitude and self-awareness.

For far too long, women's emotions have been dismissed as a weakness, something to suppress or control. But I believe your emotions are your greatest strength—your superpower. They are the compass of your soul, guiding you to deeper truths about who you are and what you need. Emotions connect you to your intuition, to others, and to something greater than yourself. They are divine messengers, shaping how you experience the world and inspiring the changes you long for. When you embrace your emotions, you embrace the fullness of life. Your emotions aren't here to hold you back; they are here to light your path. By embracing them, you can transform your life, your relationships, and your health, finding meaning and fulfillment in every moment.

## Wired to Worry

It's 10 P.M., and the fatigue of the day is weighing on you. You finally sink into the couch, Netflix on, phone in hand, savoring a rare moment of peace after a long day. Your eyelids grow heavy, but you resist the pull of sleep, because this is the only time you have for yourself. When your partner says he's heading to bed, you follow, knowing you need to wake up early for work, packing lunches, or squeezing in a morning workout. Your head hits the pillow, and you exhale, ready for rest—only for your mind to spring to life.

Suddenly, you're wide awake, your thoughts racing: *Did the kids get enough veggies today? What should I pack for lunch tomorrow? Why can't I keep up with the laundry? Should I try going vegan? I really need to wax my legs . . .* And on and on, while your partner sleeps soundly next to you. Frustrating, isn't it?

This cycle of exhaustion and sleeplessness is all too familiar for many women, leading to burnout, resentment, and constant fatigue. When we go against the natural rhythm our biology is designed for, our bodies respond with discomfort, trying to get our attention. Women are wired differently—physically, biologically, and emotionally. The more deeply we understand this, the more empowered we are to make choices that support our healing and relationships. How can we expect others to understand our struggles if we don't fully understand them ourselves? It's time to reconnect with our natural rhythm and reclaim our well-being.

Let's start with your brain. That endless "worry soup" you find yourself swimming in at night actually has a biological reason behind it. At the center of this is an area of your brain called the **anterior cingulate gyrus (ACG)**. This vital region acts as a bridge between your **limbic system**—the emotional processing center of your brain—and your **prefrontal cortex**, the part responsible for self-awareness, decision-making, planning, memory, and problem-solving. Essentially, this area governs how you regulate emotions and express yourself while analyzing your own behavior and the behavior of others.

The ACG is often referred to as the brain's "gear shifter," enabling you to move smoothly from one thought to the next and to manage tasks requiring focus and organization. In short, it's the part of your brain that keeps all the plates spinning—something every woman relies on daily to navigate life.

Interestingly, research has shown that the anterior cingulate gyrus is larger in women than in men. This means that women are biologically wired to notice the details, anticipate challenges, and worry just enough to ensure everything gets done. While this heightened connectivity is an incredible strength, it can also explain why women may feel overwhelmed or stuck in overthinking when stress or hormonal changes impact this delicate system. Understanding this connection is the first step toward shifting out of that late-night spiral.

I'm hoping that, by understanding your story and its relation to your physiology, you are now starting to realize how interconnected these two really are. The parts of your brain that help you manage your emotions and understand the world around you are impacted greatly by your story. It has been shown that childhood trauma impacts the function of the HPA axis we spoke about earlier, which controls your physical and emotional reactions to stress. Trauma and stress also impact your ACG by reducing cortical thickness and increasing neuronal loss in the region, changing how you process and express emotions, and changing how you analyze others' facial expressions, tone of voice, and social cues. In moments when others may say or do something that reminds you of your past trauma, your brain's reaction is based on the past experience and the story attached to it and creates an emotional reaction that has nothing to do with the present moment. Knowing this can help us understand our own reactions and keep the peace in our relationships!

When this area is dysregulated because of stress, it is easy to ruminate and worry and get stuck in a state of negative thoughts and behaviors, including addictions and habits that affect your health. Addictions to Netflix, social media, food, shopping, and even stress itself. This overactivity can keep you stuck in anxiety or depression, or both. Stuck in a state of worry and holding on to past hurts, not being able to see the moment for what it is but what it was. Because we have a larger ACG, we are more prone to this state of worry, and unlike men, who can shift the worry and ruminating thoughts more quickly due to their higher stores of serotonin, a calming chemical in their brains, we need to be more aware of our thoughts and patterns to prevent the cycle of destruction and to get that good night of sleep and that necessary pause before reacting.

Not only does trauma impact the connectivity between the amygdala and the prefrontal cortex, but so do hormones. There was a study done on 231 women to understand the relationship between synthetic hormones, like hormonal contraceptives, with the connectivity between the amygdala and prefrontal cortex through the functionality of the ACG. What was found was that the longer the exposure to these synthetic hormones, the less connectivity between these areas, which could result in more anxiety and less emotional regulation. This is just another example of something in your bucket of hormonal disruptors that build up over time and overflows when we don't have the right habits and tools in place to remove them as they build, leading to a storm of symptoms that seem like they have come out of nowhere.

## Finding HER Rhythm

What is rhythm? Rhythm is a pattern that creates harmony and steadiness—a sense of predictability balanced with room for change and flexibility. It's a deep-rooted knowing, a familiarity that brings safety to us and our relationships. Rhythm is the push and pull, the expansion and contraction, the inhale and exhale—movement and stillness working together. It's a dance between yin and yang, the feminine and masculine. Rhythm is play.

This play exists not only in our connections with ourselves and others but also in the intricate relationship between our neurotransmitters (our mood chemicals) and hormones. Together, they bring life and expression to our emotions, painting the colors of our experience. Throughout the month and across the stages of life, these elements move in their own rhythm.

When habits, thoughts, or stress disrupt this rhythm, we disconnect from ourselves, searching outside for answers—believing the illusion that something external will rescue or fix us. But, sister, let me tell you: The answers you seek are already dancing inside you, waiting to be unleashed.

The yin and yang cycles within you are reflections of the polarities and rhythm that exist in your emotions, thoughts, actions, and life stages. Yin and yang are present in all of us. Even as a woman, you have access to yang energy, the masculine force that brings action, drive, and strength into your day. The interplay between yin and yang—softness and strength, flexibility and structure, being and doing—is a reminder of the harmony your body and mind crave. It's when we get stuck in one state that imbalance arises, throwing us out of rhythm. When stuck in yang, the masculine energy, we can begin to wear busyness and stress like badges of honor. Life becomes an endless series of tasks, pushing us to embody a personality that thrives on aggression and constant activity just to survive. We often don't even notice how or when it happened—when we lost the ability to play and shifted into living life as if it were a race with no finish line.

Sometimes, leaning into masculine energy feels like a necessity. A single mom working tirelessly to care for her kids, a woman proving her worth in a demanding company, a mom trying to give her children everything she didn't have, or a menopausal woman stepping into new independence only to shift into caregiving for elderly parents. Sometimes, it's about staying in control of your environment and life—a response to past trauma that left you feeling unsafe and powerless. The hamster wheel never stops, and the only way to get through the day is by tapping into that masculine energy, giving you the false boost needed to push forward.

But what no one tells us is that tipping too far into the masculine for too long comes at a cost. The body begins to break down—your muscles weaken, your hair thins, your skin dulls, and your hormones falter. Chronic rushing, pleasing, and abandoning yourself keep your stress hormones in overdrive, breaking down rather than building up.

The magic lies in learning the dance between masculine and feminine energy. When you can access action and drive when needed and then return to the feminine energy of healing, growth, compassion, empathy, grace, and softness, you create harmony. It's in this balance that your hormones, neurotransmitters, and emotions can work together in a symphony that supports your well-being and allows you to truly thrive.

My patient Katie came to me after struggling for years to regulate her hormones. Her periods were unpredictable, and her emotions seemed to ride the same roller coaster. When she did bleed, it was so heavy, she had to wear a menstrual cup, a pad, and even extra layers of toilet paper to prevent leaking. The bleeding would sometimes last one to two weeks, leaving her exhausted, frustrated, and unable to catch a break. Slowing down simply wasn't an option—she had a full-time job and two kids involved in multiple activities, all of which required her constant attention. Katie was always on the go, juggling too much without a moment to pause.

When she sought help from her doctor, she was offered the usual quick fixes: birth control pills or an IUD, paired with antianxiety medication to manage her stress around her periods. But Katie had tried birth control before and hated the way it made her feel—she gained weight and felt emotionally numb and disconnected from herself. She knew there had to be another way and was ready to dig deeper to uncover why her body seemed to be crying out for help.

What finally prompted Katie to see me, despite her packed schedule, was her kids. One day, her oldest child asked her why she was always on edge and grumpy, confessing how hard it was to walk on eggshells around her because he never knew which version of "Mom" he would get that day. That conversation broke her. She realized she was slowly losing the connection with her kids that she deeply valued. On top of that, she felt completely disconnected from her husband. Every day she was running on fumes, resentful toward him without fully understanding why. Their physical relationship had dwindled, and emotionally, they felt worlds apart.

In one of our sessions, I asked her, "What do you feel you're gaining from living this way, and what do you feel like you're losing?"

Her response was raw and honest: "I'm gaining control, acknowledgment, validation, and a sense that I'm doing what I'm supposed to, but in the process, I'm losing myself and my most important relationships. I don't even know how I got here."

We ran some tests and uncovered what her body was trying to tell her. She was in a state of estrogen dominance and had fibroids in her uterus, and her adrenal

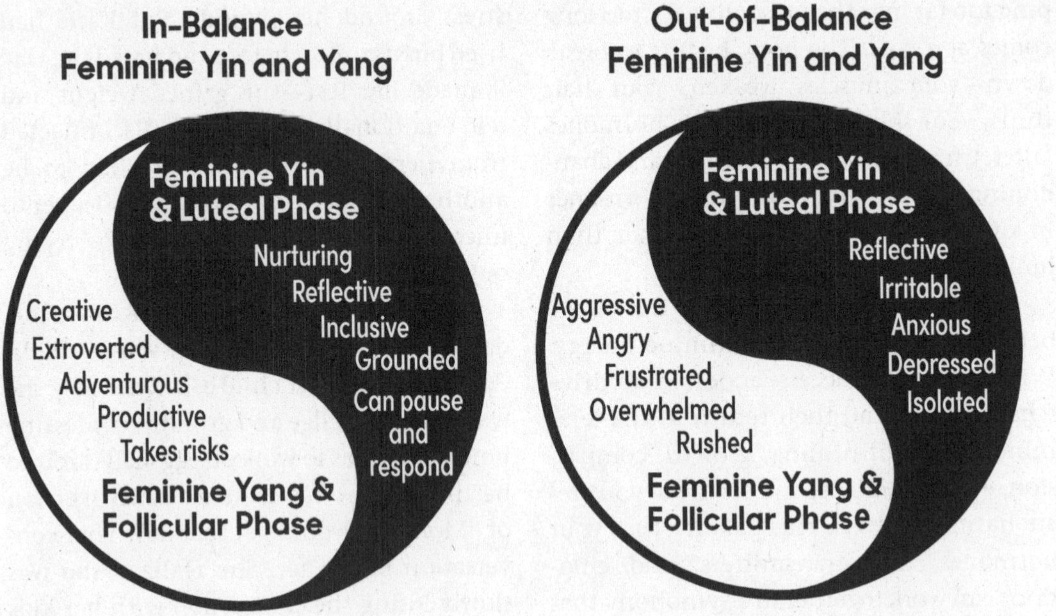


glands were completely burned-out after years of operating on overdrive. Her cortisol levels had bottomed out, her dopamine levels were low, and her thyroid was in the subclinical hypothyroid range, leaving her feeling depressed, apathetic, and stuck.

As we began working to support Katie's hormones through herbs, nutrition, and hormone therapy, her energy slowly started to return. But as her physical body healed, it became clear that the deeper work still lay ahead. True hormonal healing cannot happen without addressing the heart. My role wasn't just to guide her physically but also to help her reconnect with her heart and begin mending the broken pieces.

Katie opened up about her childhood—a time when she felt deeply unwanted. She shared how the only way she could get her parents' attention was by excelling in school and sports. She learned to stay quiet and keep busy to avoid disturbing an already chaotic household. She watched her mother endure emotional abuse in a marriage she felt trapped in because of financial dependence, leaving Katie with a front-row seat to the cost of vulnerability and dependence.

As a little girl, Katie made a silent contract with herself and the universe: She would never rely on anyone financially or emotionally, she would stay in control so she'd never be caught off guard, she would keep busy to survive, and she would never let her guard down—because letting go meant getting stuck just like her mother. These silent promises built walls around her heart, walls that served to protect her but also kept her disconnected. This identity kept her feeling safe for years, but eventually, her body and mind couldn't sustain it any longer. Her body said, "*Enough*." It was time to find herself again, to come home to herself, and to heal so she could truly be present and create a sense of home for her family.

This is a powerful example of what happens when women get stuck in their masculine energy and lose access to their natural feminine rhythm. When a woman feels the need to lead in her relationship, it's easy to default to control and competition instead of trust. Her past experiences shape her current responses, as this is how she's learned to feel safe and seen. From a young age, Katie's body had adapted by increasing cortisol, her stress hormone, while suppressing her feminine hormones like progesterone and estrogen. Over time, this had created hormonal imbalances and deepened the belief that she needed to carry everything on her own to survive.

When she began to see how the silent contract she had made with herself shaped her life, choices, and identity, she finally started her healing journey. She questioned her reactions to her husband and explored ways for him to step more into his supportive masculine energy. This allowed her to trust that she could be held and supported as she reconnected with her feminine.

Changing old habits and relationship dynamics isn't easy, but it opened an opportunity for growth—for Katie to heal and for her partner to find his role in their relationship. Her strength had often left him feeling like she didn't need him, so he had stepped back, leaving her feeling even more overwhelmed and alone. All she had wanted was for him to say, "I see you. I've got you. How can I show up for you?"

This simple shift changed everything. No longer trapped in resentment or relying on unspoken expectations, Katie allowed herself to be vulnerable and ask for what she needed. She began to melt into the softness her heart had been longing for, creating space for both of them to grow in their rhythm together.

CHAPTER 4

# Decoding Your HER Cycles

I always thought I'd have daughters—little girls I could raise to be strong and confident, to show the world, and my culture, that a woman's worth is inherent, not something she has to fight for. Growing up straddling two cultures, both Canadian and Indian, I witnessed firsthand how boys were celebrated while girls were often met with disappointment. When my brother was born, the community rejoiced with sweets and parties; when my sister arrived, there were tears. It cemented a belief in me: Being a girl wasn't enough. I prayed that in my next life, I'd be a boy, imagining the freedom they seemed to have—to go where they wanted, wear what they wanted, and simply *be*. This belief, tangled with shame and resentment, shaped so much of my identity and my choices. By the time I was 13, I felt broken, hopeless, and trapped in a body and culture I both loved and hated.

What I didn't realize then was how deeply my unprocessed pain and cultural conditioning were shaping my hormones, emotions, and future health. My period had started at 11, already shrouded in shame and secrecy. To me, menstruation became a symbol of everything that felt out of control in my life, the very thing that tied me to an identity I couldn't escape. In a desperate attempt to feel some autonomy, I deprived myself nutritionally and turned to self-harm, carving words like *I hate life* into my skin. I couldn't have known then how these choices, combined with the unhealed trauma from my childhood, were creating patterns that would impact my body, mind, and relationships as I grew into the woman I am today.

For a young woman who begins menstruating, it can take up to anywhere from a few months to seven years for menstruation to regulate and feel steady. How quickly or how long this will take is dependent on your premenarchal health nutritionally, and—I would say, most importantly—emotionally. Earlier we spoke about the HPA axis and its influence on hormones. The HPO axis, the hypothalamic-pituitary-ovarian axis, works alongside the HPA axis; these are the neuroendocrine systems that play a key role in a young woman's development and puberty. We learned that the HPA axis is influenced by stress, whether it is perceived stress, anticipatory stress, in-the-moment stress, or even imaginary and mental stress. So, one can connect the idea that if this system is overly tasked, it could in fact influence the HPO axis that is trying to regulate your hormones for regular periods.

The HPA axis contributes to the release of androgenic hormones like DHEA-S, dehydroepiandrosterone sulfate, during adrenarche—a precursor to puberty where androgen hormone production is high, which can be between ages five and eight for females, in mid-to-late childhood. Between the ages of six and seven, the adrenal glands are signaled to release DHEA-S without a rise in cortisol, your stress hormone. However, if there are events and experiences during that time that activate a rise in cortisol, it can change the expression and release of DHEA-S, as the two have an inverse relationship. If one needs to go up, the other needs to come down. Those events or experiences

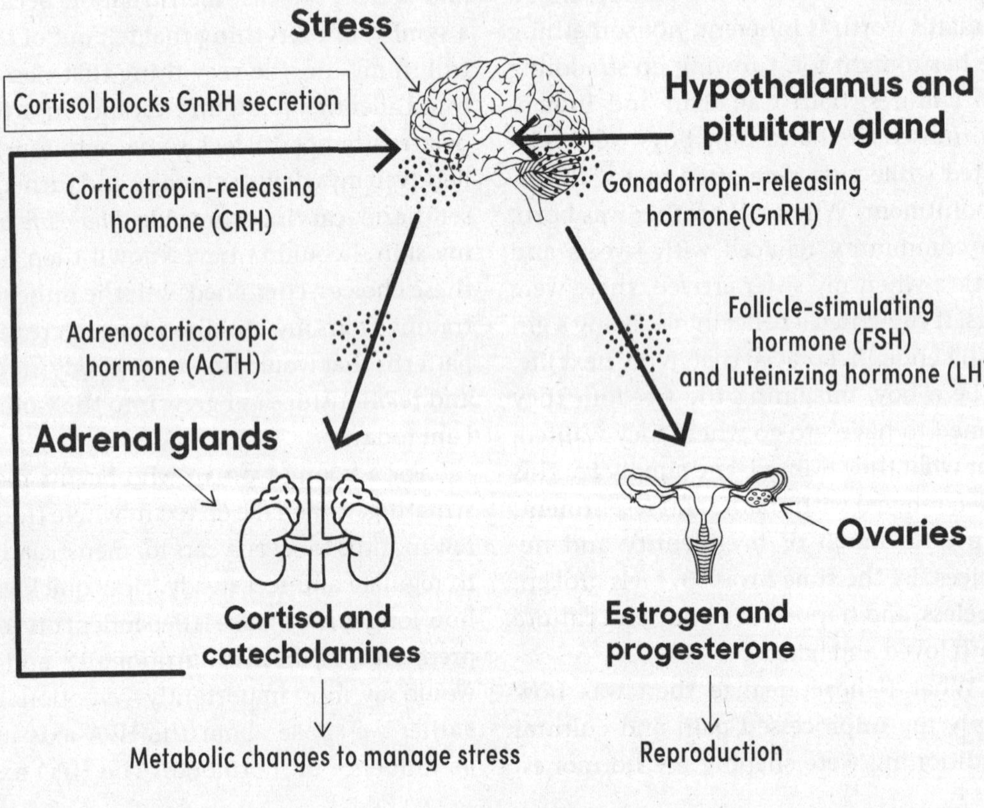

don't have to be big-T traumas like parents divorcing, abuse, or neglect; they can be a result of feeling unsafe, unwanted, and unloved in different forms from different people in your life to trigger a response of stress and survival. Your early input to your hormonal system can change according to those various moments.

Between ages 7 and 10, there is an increase in gonadotropin-releasing hormone (GnRh), released by your hypothalamus, stimulating the pituitary gland to release luteinizing hormone (LH) and follicle-stimulating hormone (FSH), all in the hopes to establish a rhythm for your ovaries and adrenals to secrete the right hormones at the right time. Like a beautiful symphony working together to create sounds that can evoke emotion, so is this dance among your neuroendocrine system and hormones to help you become tuned in to your unique song. When your body has faced stress, trauma, or emotional and nutritional deprivation, it can throw your hormones out of balance, making it harder to regulate your emotions, connect in relationships, or even understand yourself. These early experiences shape the patterns your hormonal system adopts to help you survive, creating identities and responses that may no longer serve you as an adult.

Through my own journey—navigating personal challenges like a painful divorce and hormonal chaos—I've learned that these patterns can be undone. You have the power to rewrite your story, reclaim your sense of control, and heal the wounds of your past. Healing often begins with reconnecting with your inner child—acknowledging her pain, validating her experiences, and reminding her of her strength and softness. It's about breaking down the walls around your heart and returning to yourself with love and compassion.

For me, this process deepened when I embraced the balance of feminine yin and yang energies. It began during the births of my two sons, where I witnessed the harmony of strength and surrender needed to bring life into the world. Whether birthing a child, an idea, or a dream, we are vessels of creation—a union of yin and yang, masculine and feminine energies.

As parents, my husband and I strive to teach our boys about this balance through our relationship. We are their first models of feminine and masculine energy. Though imperfect, we aim to show them how relationships—whether with ourselves, others, or the divine—evolve through effort, understanding, and healing.

Your hormones mirror this interplay. Estrogen works in harmony with progesterone; neurotransmitters like serotonin and gamma-aminobutyric acid (GABA) rely on these hormones to help you feel calm and balanced, while dopamine depends on testosterone to bring joy and motivation. Just as relationships outside your body require nurturing to thrive, so do the relationships within. Understanding these connections—what disrupts them and what supports them—is the first step in your journey to healing and self-discovery. Let's explore the roles your hormones play in shaping your emotions, personality, and relationships, and how they can guide you toward a more balanced and fulfilled life.

## Getting to Know Your Hormonal Archetypes

As a woman with a natural menstrual cycle, your emotional and physical states shift noticeably week by week. It can feel like juggling multiple personalities as your hormones rise and fall, influencing not only your mood but also how you respond to emotions and the world around you. Layer in the effects of past trauma and ongoing stress, and you have a recipe for what can feel like an unpredictable storm that seems to come out of nowhere.

For women in perimenopause, this experience can feel even more destabilizing, as fluctuating estrogen levels send them on a hormonal roller coaster. Meanwhile, postmenopausal women who have moved beyond these shifts might still face uncertainty with their body and mind, particularly if they transitioned into menopause with low hormone levels. Without these hormonal "buffers," emotions and unresolved past hurts that may have been previously buried often rise to the surface, demanding attention and healing.

Many women notice that their emotions feel particularly unstable during the luteal phase—the second half of the menstrual cycle following ovulation. Research supports this observation. A review highlights those women with a history of trauma or post-traumatic stress disorder (PTSD) experience heightened psychological stress and PTSD symptoms during the late luteal phase. This phase is marked by a sharp decline in estrogen and progesterone levels, signaling the body to prepare for menstruation. These hormonal drops seem to leave

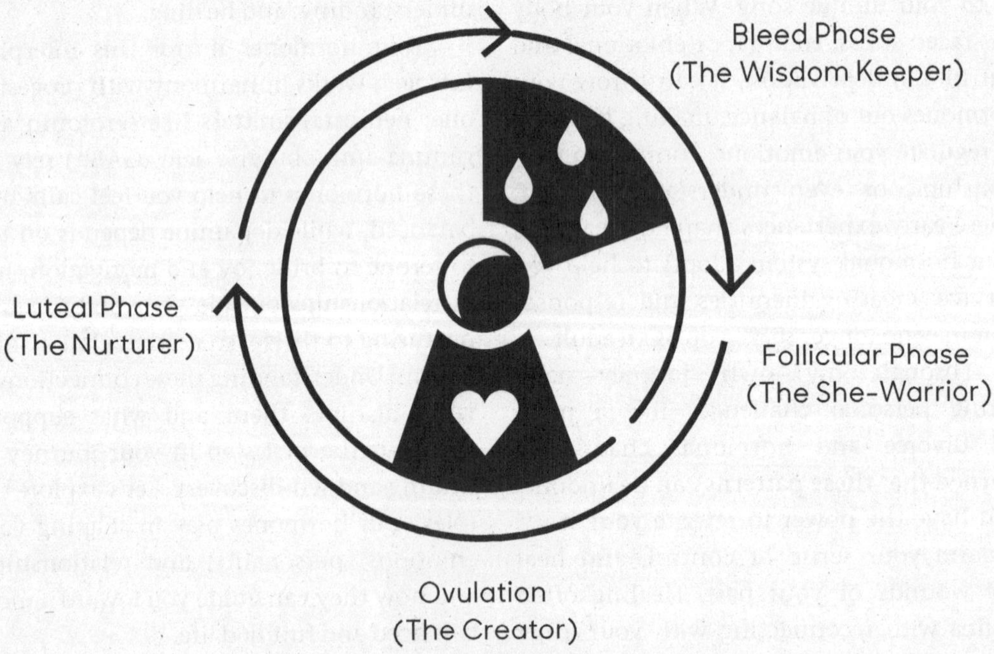

the nervous system more vulnerable, reducing its ability to cope with stress effectively.

One study measured alpha-amylase, an enzyme linked to stress, in saliva and found that levels of this enzyme were significantly elevated in the late luteal phase. This contrasts with a blunted response during the follicular phase, when estrogen levels are higher. Elevated alpha-amylase levels are associated with heightened sympathetic nervous system activity—commonly referred to as the "fight, flight, freeze, or please" response—which explains why stress may feel magnified during this time.

These findings help illuminate why the premenstrual week can feel overwhelming. Many women report mood swings, increased sensitivity, and emotional outbursts—crying over a commercial, feeling irritable, or reacting intensely to minor comments. It seems our bodies are designed to slow down and destress in preparation for releasing not only physical tissue but also emotional "baggage" from the month. Yet, modern culture often pushes us to ignore these natural rhythms, forcing us to power through rather than honor this time of introspection and renewal.

The emotional ups and downs of your cycle can feel overwhelming, especially when you notice a pattern but don't understand how to break free from it. These symptoms—mood swings, irritability, or heightened sensitivity—are more than random reactions; they are signals, revealing pieces of your past and present that influence your emotional and physical state. Understanding this connection can empower you to reclaim control, but for some women, especially those with premenstrual dysphoric disorder (PMDD), the challenge can feel insurmountable.

Women with PMDD face unique biological hurdles. Research shows they have reduced levels of allopregnanolone, a metabolite of progesterone crucial for regulating GABA, a neurotransmitter responsible for calmness during stress. Without sufficient GABA activity, women with PMDD may experience heightened agitation and reactivity, leading to miscommunications and strained relationships. These challenges are compounded by disruptions in the HPA axis, the system that governs cortisol production. Women with PMDD often experience a delayed cortisol awakening response, with their cortisol levels rising 15 minutes later than expected. This delay can result in sluggish mornings, low energy, and diminished motivation, setting a frustrating tone for the day.

To make matters more complex, women with PMDD who have a history of trauma show increased reactivity in beta-1 and beta-2 adrenoreceptors, critical components of the stress response. This heightened sensitivity amplifies the body's reaction to even minor stressors, intensifying emotional volatility during both the follicular and luteal phases.

But why do these shifts occur? Why are cortisol responses blunted, allopregnanolone levels low, and stress receptors more reactive? The answer often lies in a combination of chronic stress, encompassing physical, emotional, and chemical stressors.

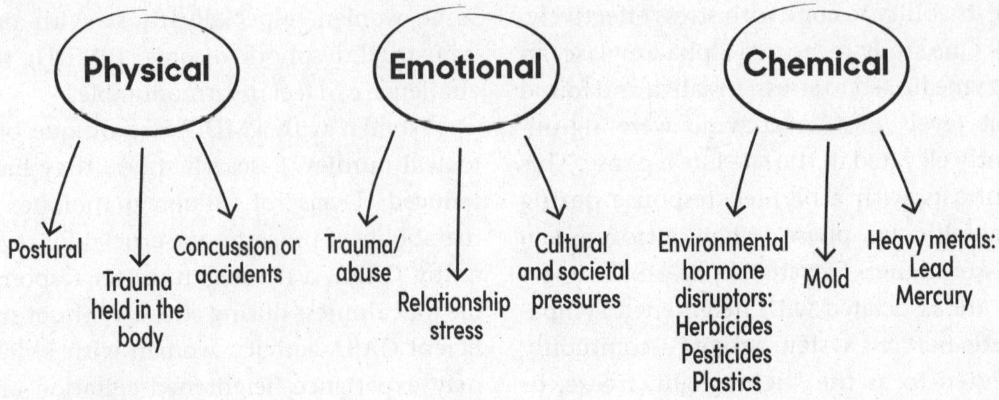


By recognizing these factors and addressing the underlying stress, it becomes possible to disrupt these cycles, helping women find relief and restore balance.

What I have seen in the women I work with is this sense of hopelessness when they cannot get a handle on how they feel or understand why they feel that way. My job has always been to restore their hope by showing them, "This isn't who you are, it is how your body and brain have decided to respond to keep you safe from the stressors." As I help them step into safety and begin the process of trusting their bodies, they can then begin the process of redefining their relationship with themselves. How they feel is no longer a burden but a gift that helps them see the truth behind the veil of protection. When they begin to see the elements of the past and present environments that have shaped their hormonal story, we can take time to release the charge of the triggers in their lives to rebuild and reclaim the power that was given away.

Each phase of your cycle brings subtle shifts that can influence how you approach life. The charts on the next page illustrate these shifts, showing what they look like when your hormones are in balance versus when stressors have altered your hormonal and neuronal pathways.

The menstrual cycle is a dynamic process that shifts both hormonally and emotionally across its four phases, each with distinct physical markers and dominant hormones. Understanding these phases helps illuminate how hormonal balance—or imbalance—impacts your well-being.

The follicular phase—the phase I call the She-Warrior—begins on the first day of your period and lasts until ovulation. During this time, estrogen gradually rises as the body prepares to mature an egg. Physically, this phase is defined by the thickening of the uterine lining in preparation for potential pregnancy. When hormones are balanced, you may feel confident, decisive, energized, and outgoing, as estrogen supports mental clarity and physical vitality. However, imbalances can lead to hyperactivity, indecision, or a sense of low mood, manifesting as feelings of being rushed or apathetic.

Ovulation—the Creator—is the shortest phase of the cycle, lasting about 24 to 48 hours, and occurs when the mature egg is released from the ovary. Testosterone and oxytocin peak during this phase, enhancing feelings of connection, creativity, and motivation. Physically, this phase is characterized by cervical mucus changes, often becoming clear and stretchy, indicating fertility. In balance, these hormones make you feel vibrant, confident, and deeply connected to others. When out of balance, however, you might experience feelings of rigidity, mistrust, or hopelessness, along with physical tension.

The luteal phase—the Nurturer—spans approximately 10 to 14 days after ovulation, dominated by a rise in progesterone, which helps maintain a potential pregnancy. Physically, your body shifts toward preparation for menstruation if pregnancy does not occur, and you may notice increased body temperature or breast tenderness, among other changes. When progesterone is balanced, this phase brings calmness, self-awareness, and a natural desire to rest and reflect. However, hormonal imbalances can trigger anxiety, fear, rage, or self-doubt, making it challenging to maintain emotional stability.

The menstrual phase—the Wisdom Keeper—begins when hormone levels, particularly estrogen and progesterone, drop significantly, causing the uterine lining to shed. Physically, this is marked by menstruation, which can last three to seven days and is a deep detoxification process. When hormones are balanced, this phase

**Follicular Phase States and Emotions**

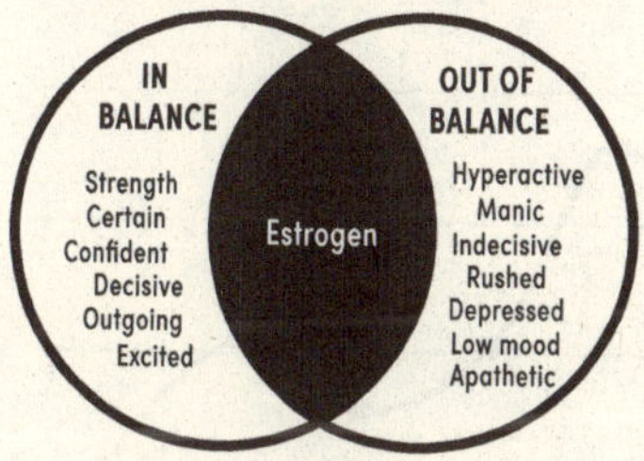


**Ovulation Phase States and Emotions**

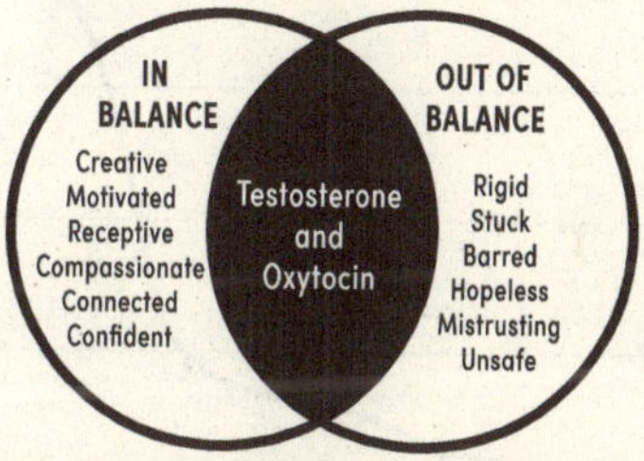


**Luteal Phase States and Emotions**

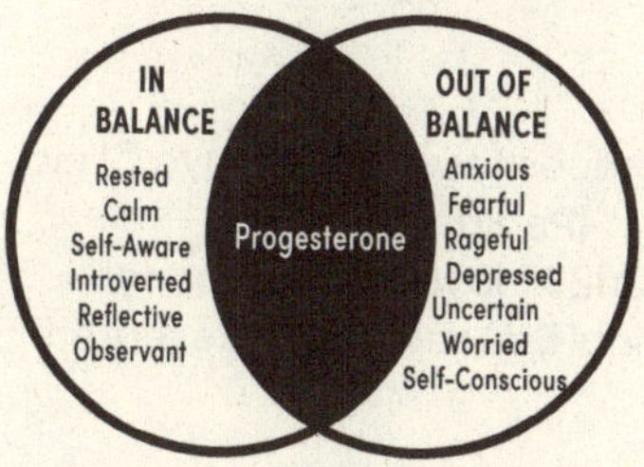


**Bleed Phase States and Emotions**

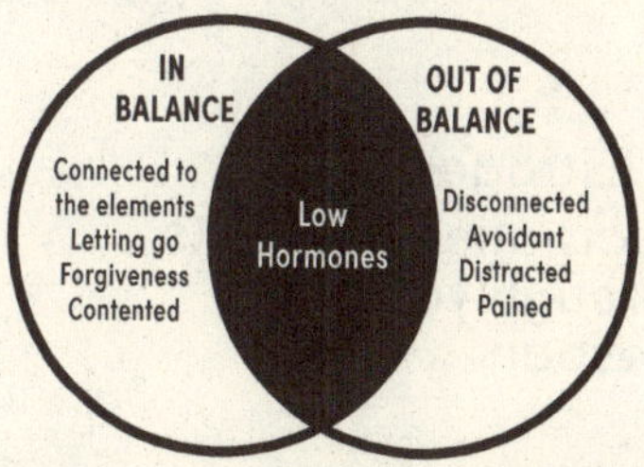

fosters a sense of release, forgiveness, and contentment, as the body resets for a new cycle. In contrast, imbalances can lead to feelings of disconnection, avoidance, or distraction, along with painful cramps or heavy bleeding.

Each phase of the cycle offers unique insights into your body's needs and rhythms. By understanding the hormonal and physical shifts that define each stage, you can better support your health and understand the emotional shifts you may be experiencing. There are so many interconnections between how you think, what you feel, and how your body responds with various hormones and neurochemicals. There are also many things happening behind the scenes in your brain and nervous system that dictate those relationships between the hormones that carry the messages and the neurotransmitters that help you experience them through your emotional states. Let's take a deeper dive into each hormone and its connected neurochemical and nutrient families to better understand how we can support their relationship so you can support yours!

## Estrogen—HER Radiance

We all need her. That one person that cheers you on and helps you get up when you are feeling down. What if I told you she already exists in you and has been just waiting for you to unleash her potential? Estrogen, the vivacious virago, the sister that is the life of

### Estrogen Fluctuations

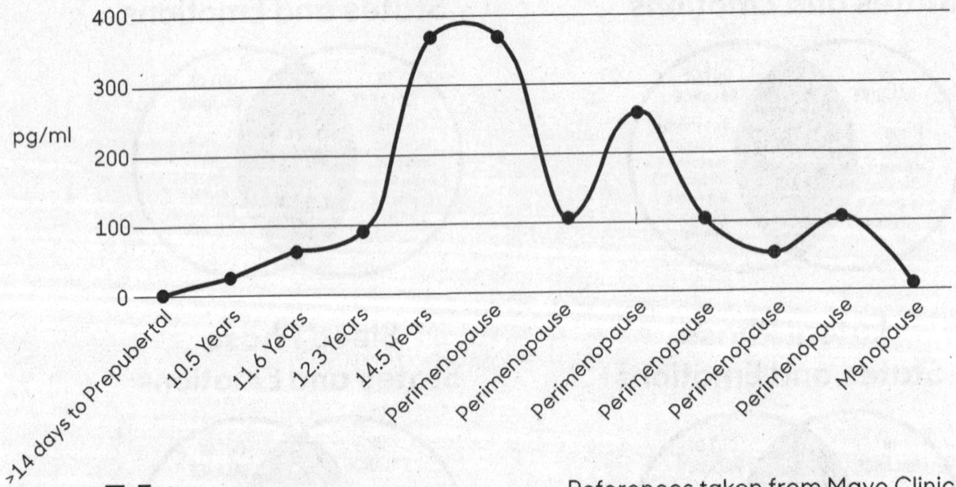


■ Estrogen fluctuating amounts through your lifespan

References taken from Mayo Clinic Pediatric Catalog ©2023 Mayo Foundation for Medical Education and Research

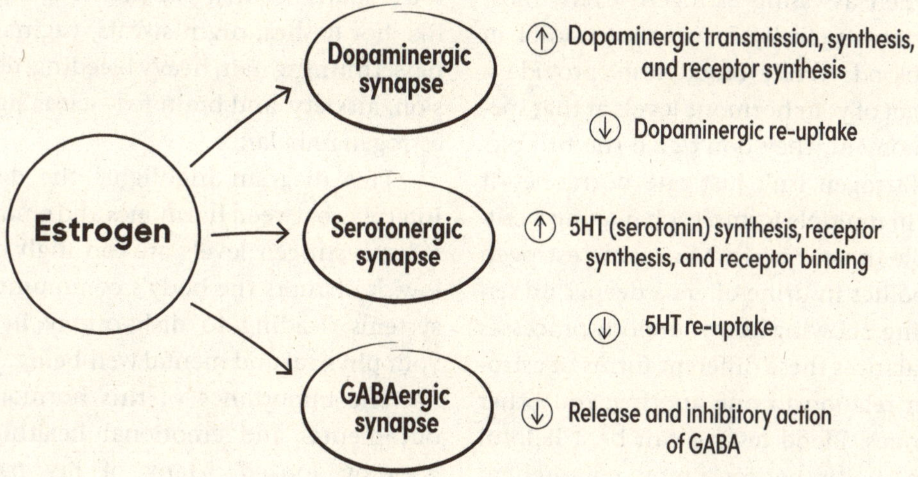


the party and has no bounds, is constantly rooting for you by creating connections in your brain and vitality in your body. You have three forms of estrogen: estradiol (the party starter), estrone (the rebel), and estriol (the creative). Estradiol is the dominant estrogen in your reproductive years, while estrone is made continuously even after menopause by your adrenal glands and fat tissue. Estrone can convert into estradiol when needed and stores your estrogen (you know that pesky weight gain around the belly is all thanks to this one when she isn't following the rules and stays in storing mode instead of converting!). Estriol is mostly active during pregnancy and can be used in bioidentical hormone therapy along with estradiol to help reduce symptoms like hot flashes, night sweats, and vaginal dryness.

When estradiol is produced by the dominant ovarian follicle and rises in the follicular phase, the emotional changes that occur in that phase give rise to optimism, confidence, and motivation. You know that feeling—right when you are about to finish your bleed, and all of a sudden, you are seeing more color in your world, you're starting to notice what is working in your life rather than focusing on what isn't, and that time where the loud chewing sounds your husband makes seem to fade into the background, well, that is estrogen reminding you of your awesomeness! Estrogen can be connected to feeling extremely grounded and steady while excited and happy.

Many women with low estrogen levels report experiencing more depression, anxiety, and an overall sense of "blah." This is because estrogen plays a key role in your brain's ability to use neurotransmitters like dopamine and serotonin—both essential for feeling motivated and happy. Think of estrogen as the "juiciness" your body thrives on: It hydrates your skin, thickens your hair, and strengthens your bones. When estrogen levels drop, it's as if that vitality is drained from every cell, leaving you feeling dry, brittle, and emotionally depleted.

When assessing estrogen levels, most physicians typically focus on estradiol in your blood. While blood tests provide a snapshot of your hormone levels at that specific moment, they don't give the full picture. Estrogen isn't just one hormone—it exists in multiple forms, each playing a critical role in your body. Measuring estrogen metabolites in urine offers a deeper understanding, showing how your body processes and balances these different forms of estrogen in relation to one another and other hormones. Blood testing can be a helpful starting point, but for a more comprehensive view, urine testing is often the way to go. In the chapters ahead, we'll explore this in more detail. Below is an overview of how estrogen levels in the blood shift throughout your life as you age.

Postmenopause, estrogen levels drop significantly, but the real challenge often begins in the perimenopause phase. During this transition, estrogen fluctuates wildly, creating a sense of imbalance just as you're navigating changes in your body and life roles. Many women experience symptoms like hot flashes, night sweats, vaginal dryness, thinning hair, heavy bleeding, depression, anxiety, and brain fog—clear signs of estrogen imbalance.

This diagram highlights the delicate interplay between hormones and emotions. When estrogen levels are too high or too low, it disrupts the body's communication systems, leading to disharmony in both your physical and mental well-being.

The importance of this hormone for our mental and emotional health often goes overlooked. Many of my patients have shared their frustration after visiting doctors, describing challenges like difficulty focusing, a lack of motivation, new and overwhelming anxiety, and even feeling these struggles throughout their entire body. Too often, the only solutions offered are medications—antidepressants, sleeping pills, or birth control—without any consideration of how hormonal imbalances might be contributing to their state.

| EFFECTS OF HIGH ESTROGEN | EFFECTS OF LOW ESTROGEN |
|---|---|
| Fibroids | Dry skin and hair |
| Polycystic ovarian syndrome | Vaginal dryness |
| Endometriosis | Hot flashes |
| Cystic acne | Night sweats |
| Anxiety | Brain fog |
| Water retention | Urinary incontinence |
| Bloating and weight gain around belly | Depression |
| Breast tenderness | Short-term memory issues |
| High sex hormone-binding globulin (therefore low testosterone) | Osteoporosis |

Estrogen is all about connection. It connects neuronal pathways in your brain, creating new pathways so you can remember important moments, so you can focus on tasks, so you can have access to neurochemicals that help you feel on purpose and in joy. She affirms how important you are, how worthy you are, and how much value you have to give to this world. Without her there is a darkness that sweeps the brain that informs the mind of unworthiness and hopelessness. This impacts how you see yourself and everyone around you. Especially those closest to you.

## Testosterone—HER Spark

Have you ever noticed that at certain times in your cycle, your partner seems extra irresistible? Or maybe there are moments when a brilliant idea strikes, and you feel a surge of energy to bring it to life. Or perhaps you wake up some mornings buzzing with excitement for the day ahead. That's the magic of testosterone, your personal motivator. While many think of this hormone as "just for men," it plays a crucial role in women too. Without testosterone, the zest for life—the spark that helps you push through challenges or bounce back from a tough day—would feel out of reach.

For women, testosterone is all about balance. Too much can lead to aggression and difficulty managing emotions, while too little can feel like depression or a loss of hope. Unfortunately, like other steroid hormones, testosterone declines as we age. By around age 25, its gradual decrease begins, but how quickly it falls is often influenced by the choices we make along the way.

For years my kid's school had a program called "grandfriends," where their class would go visit care homes once a month to do an activity with the elderly. This one day a woman from the care home was talking to the children about what to expect and how excited the residents were to see all of them. She then posed a question to the kids—now, these are five-year-olds: "What happens when you get old?"

Here are some of the answers: "You can't walk anymore," "Your muscles are gone," "You can't remember anything," "Your teeth fall out," "You get sick"—and they went on and on while I sat there, amused and disturbed by their answers all at once. This is the narrative and picture we have sold to our children, that getting old means losing who you are and living in a body that betrays you while it starts falling apart. The children are not the only ones that have been stuck in this illusion, we, too, have bought into it. Yes, things change, but how quickly and how painfully is still in our control.

The definition and strength in your muscles decline as you age because of the rapid decline in testosterone. By the time you hit menopause, 50 percent of your testosterone is gone, and for those women that must undergo a complete hysterectomy, there is a 70 percent decline in testosterone within 24 hours! Talk about a major mojo buster! Testosterone isn't just about aggression (yes, it can be when it is too high); it is about strength, drive, and mood enhancement, and it allows you to feel a sense of purpose.

There's a common assumption that when it comes to testosterone, more is always better—especially if you're noticing its impact on your intimacy and connection with your partner. But like everything in the body, balance is key. Testosterone naturally peaks just before and during ovulation for menstruating women and is often lower in menopausal women. This is why finding ways to optimize the levels you do have is so important.

There's also a misconception that women should always feel desire for their partner or that intimacy should come effortlessly. The truth is, that's not how it works. Desire can ebb and flow with hormonal changes, stress, and life's demands. It doesn't mean intimacy is out of reach—it just means you may need to create the right conditions to help you connect and get into the mood. With understanding and support, this can feel less like a challenge and more like a natural part of your rhythm.

To begin healing your relationship with testosterone, it's important to reflect on your story and the stressors that have shaped your hormonal health. One of the biggest disruptors of testosterone is high levels of a protein in the blood called sex hormone-binding globulin (SHBG). SHBG binds to testosterone, making it unavailable for your cells to use, which leads to mood disorders, low libido, and even vaginal dryness. Women with PCOS usually have low levels of SHBG, making testosterone too available and leading to symptoms like unwanted hair growth. This confirms that hormonal healing is nuanced, each one playing a particular role, and too much or too little of anything takes us off our balance.

Several factors can increase SHBG levels. One major culprit is the birth control pill. Many generations of the pill are made with synthetic testosterone, and the rise in estrogen caused by some pills signals your body to produce more SHBG, effectively reducing the free testosterone available. Other contributors include high levels of stress, which disrupt hormonal balance and increase cortisol, chronic inflammation, insulin resistance, and thyroid dysfunction. A diet low in protein or healthy fats can also play a role, as these nutrients are essential for hormone production and regulation. As we

| EFFECTS OF HIGH TESTOSTERONE | EFFECTS OF LOW TESTOSTERONE |
|---|---|
| Acne | Osteoporosis |
| Aggression | Low sex drive |
| Frustration | Low motivation |
| Polycystic ovarian syndrome | Low lean muscle mass |
| Hirsutism (male pattern hair growth in women) | Dyspareunia (painful sexual intercourse) |
| Depression | Depression |

age, a process called aromatization—where androgens like testosterone are converted into estrogen—increases, making testosterone even less available, especially in cases of weight gain, stress, and low insulin sensitivity. If you've been on the pill or have any of these contributing factors and feel disconnected from your spark, energy, or even the sexiness you once felt with your partner, you're not alone. It's not just in your head—your hormones and SHBG levels are directly influencing how you feel and function.

Testosterone isn't just about sex drive—it's a key hormone that impacts your mood, energy, and overall sense of joy through its influence on your brain and neurochemicals like serotonin and dopamine. When it's low, feelings of sadness, depression, and apathy can take over, making it hard to get out of bed or find excitement in the things you love. To cope, you might turn to external sources like food, alcohol, shopping, or even stress and chaos to feel something—anything—different from the emptiness. But this reliance on outside "fixes" can create a cycle of addiction and disconnection from yourself and others.

When joy and contentment feel out of reach, it's common to expect a partner, children, friends, or even a job to fill that void. But the truth is, you're not broken. Your body is simply missing the hormonal balance needed to feel whole. Understanding and addressing what's keeping you from accessing those emotions is the first step toward reclaiming your connection to yourself and your wholeness.

If you've ever felt the need to suppress parts of yourself growing up—like being competitive, outspoken, or using anger to create change—your brain likely got the message that it wasn't safe to express these traits. Maybe you were told "nice girls don't compete" or "keep your opinions to yourself," or perhaps someone dismissed you when you tried to share your thoughts. Each of these moments conditioned you to hide your testosterone-driven traits—your inner yang energy—creating beliefs and patterns in your brain and nervous system that it's safer to stay small and avoid making others uncomfortable.

This suppression doesn't just affect your confidence; it impacts your hormones too. In the short term, testosterone may spike during moments of internal rage or aggression, but over time, chronic suppression can lead to depletion. Testosterone, like all hormones, helps you access parts of yourself that are essential for growth and fulfillment. Supporting your hormonal health is key to breaking free from patterns of hiding and seeking external validation, allowing you to fully express who you are.

## Progesterone—HER Worthiness and Belonging

Progesterone peaks during the luteal phase, and with it, so does GABA—the neurotransmitter that promotes calm and relaxation in your brain and body—as allopregnanolone (a metabolite of progesterone) activates GABA receptors. Think of progesterone as a warm, protective layer for your nervous system—it literally helps form the myelin sheath around your nerves, the insulation your body needs to function optimally.

When that layer is depleted, as seen in conditions like postpartum depression or multiple sclerosis (both connected to low hormone levels), the effects ripple through your entire system. Sleep suffers, stress feels insurmountable, emotional regulation falters, and inflammation rises.

So, why are so many women struggling during this phase? The answer lies in one word: stress. Stress disrupts this intricate balance, stealing the calm and connection that progesterone is meant to provide. It's time to reclaim this phase as a time for rest, reflection, and reconnection.

Progesterone is a precursor to cortisol, your stress hormone. When you're stuck in a state of hypervigilance and stress, your body prioritizes producing cortisol to help you cope. To do this, it converts progesterone into cortisol, leaving less of this calming, protective hormone available to support you. Over time, this depletion can lead to burnout and heightened inflammation. That feeling like you're getting sick right before your period. The restless nights, the migraine that lifts as soon as your period starts, or the sudden waves of irritation or rage directed at your partner. All of these are signs of dysregulated progesterone, leaving you feeling like you're unraveling.

For many women, it's as if a switch flips once they begin bleeding. In the days leading up to their period, everything can feel dark and overwhelming. Thoughts turn heavy, as if nothing in life is going right, and motivation to do anything disappears. It feels like the despair will never end. But once the bleeding begins, something shifts. The body releases, the mind exhales, and suddenly it's possible to see clearly again, to feel lighter and more hopeful.

This phase, while challenging, is also an opportunity. It's a time to reflect and ask yourself: *What beliefs, pain, grief, or patterns am I holding on to that no longer serve me?* When you notice recurring thoughts, feelings, or behaviors during this time, they're often signals calling for your attention. These moments aren't about falling apart—they're about uncovering the parts of yourself or your life that need healing, giving you the chance to release what's weighing you down and move forward with greater clarity and strength.

If we understood the importance of progesterone earlier in life, we might make

| EFFECTS OF HIGH PROGESTERONE | EFFECTS OF LOW PROGESTERONE |
|---|---|
| Bloating | Hot flashes |
| Agitation | Low sex drive |
| Anxiety | Anxiety/Mood disorders |
| Fatigue | Irregular cycles |
| Vaginal dryness | Infertility/Miscarriages |
| Depression | Insomnia |

different choices—or at least realize why certain habits leave us feeling out of sync. Sure, as teens we might still choose to eat junk food, stay up all night, or skip workouts because it feels good in the moment, but at least we'd know the impact those choices have on our hormones. Today, so many young women are being diagnosed with conditions like PCOS, endometriosis, PMDD, and polyps—nearly all of which are linked to low or imbalanced progesterone.

Somewhere along the way, progesterone's value got diminished in favor of convenience. When you've had to quiet your voice, make yourself small to feel safe, or bend over backward to keep the peace, your progesterone hides right along with you. This hormone thrives when you feel safe, calm, and supported. But in a world that rarely nurtures those states, we suppress not only our voices but the very hormone that helps regulate our cycles, soothe our emotions, and keep us balanced.

Pain and luteal-phase symptoms are not normal—they're just something we've been conditioned to live with. These symptoms are your body's way of signaling that something deeper needs attention. It could be a mineral deficiency, a structural issue, or perhaps your progesterone isn't getting the support it needs to rise during the luteal phase to keep things balanced. I often invite my patients to reflect on their themes of discomfort during this time. Ask yourself, *Am I having the same argument with my partner every single month? Are the same negative thoughts consuming my mind?* If so, you can ask—*What do I need to change in my life, need to heal, or need to understand?* You may learn exactly what you need to change your luteal experience. As you begin to voice your concerns with your partner before the resentment sets in or begin to set your boundaries to make sure you give your body time to rest from the chaos, you may find those luteal trends or themes start to change.

What amazes me is how easily our society accepts masking these issues with a pill just to keep up with the chaos and busyness of modern life. But the pain you feel is not random—it's your body trying to tell you a story. The growths, the heavy bleeding, the irritability, and the anxiety are all pieces of that story, and it's in the luteal phase, when progesterone is supposed to take the lead, that the imbalance speaks the loudest. Isn't it time we start listening?

Grandmother energy. This is the essence of progesterone—the nurturing, calming force that helps you feel steady in both your emotional and physical body. This is its true nature, just as it is yours. Ideally, your luteal phase should be a time when you feel calm, intuitive, present, and deeply connected to yourself—a time to anchor in your worth. Yet, for so many women, it feels like the complete opposite. Instead of peace, they experience fear, frustration, and discomfort, overshadowed by the symptoms of imbalance.

After giving birth to our second son when I was 35 years old, I noticed a huge shift in my hormones. I would dread my luteal phase, knowing I was going to feel bloated, depressed, on edge, and have even more sleepless nights. I could feel a change as soon as I would ovulate and then a switch back to normal as soon as I would bleed.

It was getting to the point where everything my husband did was wrong and my patience for my boys was so low that I had to give myself time-outs in the bathroom so I wouldn't overreact when they were just being kids.

After some testing it was clear that my progesterone was low, and I needed to restore it ASAP! I took some herbs, started some nutrient IV therapy, made yoga and meditation a priority, and did some bioidentical progesterone—and it was like my body and mind could finally exhale. I remember the first few days of using the progesterone. It was like I was flooded with warmth and calm, and I realized that this was the switch my patients were talking about all along! Now, not everyone has the same experience, and using hormones is very nuanced and is specific to the individual. For me, I had found the right amount and the right combination of lifestyle and nutrition factors that gave me the relief I needed, and the perspective shift I desperately needed, to feel steadier and more grounded for my family. As the years went on and I became more and more tuned in to my hormones and started the healing I needed around my past traumas and stresses, I had finally found a hormonal groove and rhythm that worked. My periods were regular, moods were stable, and everything felt like I was moving in the right direction, and then I turned 42.

In traditional Chinese medicine, because women carry the yin energy, it is said that women move through seven-year cycles in their bodies, especially in relation to the reproductive system. At the age of 42, I was entering my sixth cycle, and according to *The Yellow Emperor's Classic of Internal*

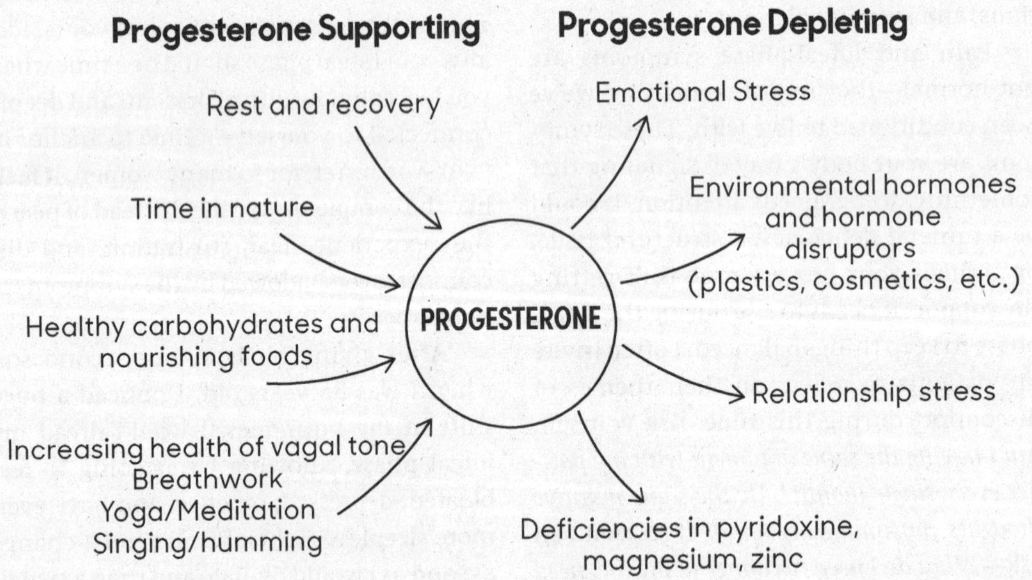

*Medicine,* a Chinese medical text, women in this stage are dealing with weak yang channels, their face darkens, and hair turns gray, basically saying they enter the stage of saggy skin, low vitality, and loss of everything! A lot changed for me in this stage: my recovery time, my moods, my weight distribution, and for the first time I said hello to saggy skin on the backs of my arms. Let's just say it didn't feel amazing, and I also knew it was an opportunity to change the narrative. We will uncover more about this stage in the coming chapters, but what was super clear here was that I had to protect my progesterone and all my hormones, no matter what. For me, this translated to self-care, now more than ever, was essential and nonnegotiable.

Safeguarding your progesterone is one of the best ways to ensure your mental, emotional, and physical well-being. I would venture to say, your spiritual well-being as well. In a spiritual practice, we learn to listen, to connect, and to realize the vastness of our universe and ourselves. We see the connection in all things and realize the light that we see in others reflects the light we carry within ourselves. It is often in moments of pain and suffering that we look toward God, source, the universe for answers and comfort. This time in our cycle gives us that same opportunity. An opportunity to pause and ask for help, for guidance, and for deeper understanding of us to help put the pieces back together, as we uncover the truth behind it all, that the answers are already within. When we are far away from our spirit and abandoning our soul through acts of violence toward ourselves through the choices we make, when we are far away and disconnected from our bodies and lost in the noise of who we are supposed to be, that is when we move further away from spirit and further away from healing. It is when we can see that all we must do is make a choice to nurture and understand ourselves and see the brilliance of this human design, where our soul gets to take form and experience life, that is when the healing at all levels begins.

## Oxytocin—HER Connection

The smell of a baby, the juicy secrets between you and your girlfriends as a child, the whole-body orgasm, the warm hug from your grandmother—what creates the feeling of euphoria during these moments is your neurohormone oxytocin. That feeling that wraps its arms around you is a feeling of acceptance, love, compassion, and connection; that flood of oxytocin in your system is telling you everything is safe, and everything is going to be okay. Often called the love hormone, oxytocin is a reminder that we humans are wired for connection and thrive in safety. It helps build trust. Trust within yourself and trust in the world around you. During puberty, estrogen increases the production of oxytocin, encouraging a young woman toward social bonding. Intimacy helps increase its production, and its increased production seeks out more intimacy. During ovulation, oxytocin, alongside the neurotransmitter dopamine, rises, increasing that desire to connect. Connection doesn't always have to be physical: It's in conversation, it's in sitting with your girlfriends and laughing, it's in getting together and doing a group yoga class. This hormone and desire to bond with others is especially high in your teens, correlating with higher amounts of estrogen. When estrogen drops in menopause, so can oxytocin, leading to those feelings of loneliness that so many women in menopause describe.

One of the greatest blocks to this hormone is trauma and stress. Under chronic stress, its production decreases, but interestingly, in acute stress, its production increases to help bring cortisol back to its prestress baseline. To help calm the body down and to convey to the brain that all is well and that the stress was just temporary. Now, this is a hormone that needs to be bottled up and given to every woman out there! However, it isn't that simple. Some studies have shown that giving oxytocin to those who have had PTSD or severe trauma creates more anxiety and stress. So, as we can see with all the other hormones, this, too, needs a nuanced approach when dealing with chronic stress and a history of trauma. When you have had to deal with childhood adversity, your ability to produce oxytocin is lowered, leaving you more reactive and less resilient in your responses to stress. Not only does your ability to manage stress go down but so does self-confidence and your capacity to trust.

A woman came to me some time ago who couldn't understand why she was so full of rage. She had a family she loved, a job that fulfilled her, and a husband that supported her. But more often than not, especially around ovulation, she felt this feeling of rage and like she was about to implode. Her husband was complaining that she was snapping at him even in public and had no patience for the kids. He was quick to remind her that when they were younger, she never seemed to be bothered by the clothes on the floor, the long days of golfing, and the forgetting of important dates, but now, instead of staying in silence, she spoke up every time and in a way that was often followed by conflict. She found her voice and wasn't going to give it up. It felt good to finally say everything she was thinking and at the same time knew how she was saying it was creating chaos in the family.

When we began working together, it became clear that she had spent most of her life trying to please everyone around her. This pattern was rooted in her childhood, where neglect and unpredictability shaped her responses. Sharing her needs or emotions often led to conflict or stress in her parents, so she learned to stay quiet, believing that keeping the peace was the only way to feel safe. The volatility in her home made her constantly walk on eggshells, unable

| EFFECTS OF HIGH OXYTOCIN | EFFECTS OF LOW OXYTOCIN |
|---|---|
| Strengthens bad memories | Irritability/Insomnia |
| Dysmenorrhea | Lack of joy |
| Anxiety and fear for future triggers connected to past bad social experiences | Hard to reach orgasm or be affectionate |

to trust her environment or her ability to maintain harmony. This survival mechanism followed her into adulthood, showing up in her relationships, where she prioritized her partner's needs over her own and silenced her voice.

Then perimenopause hit, and it was like a floodgate of truth opened. The fluctuations in her estrogen and a decline in oxytocin brought suppressed emotions to the surface, with rage and frustration demanding to be heard. The changing balance between testosterone and estrogen left her feeling aggressive and assertive at times, followed by guilt and regret. These emotional highs and lows left her feeling out of control and disconnected from herself and her loved ones.

To help her step off this roller coaster, we focused on increasing her oxytocin—the hormone of connection and trust—through simple, intentional practices that nurtured her sense of safety and joy. We also explored techniques to rebuild trust in herself and those around her. By balancing her hormones and addressing the deeper roots of her emotional reactions, she was able to set healthy boundaries and communicate her needs effectively. This work not only transformed her relationship with herself but also strengthened her bonds with her kids and her partner, creating a life where her voice was no longer silenced but celebrated.

## The Thyroid—HER Voice

There is a time in a woman's life where it can feel like she just can't get a break. With aging parents that need her constant support to help them navigate their health, kids needing her constant attention, a career that feels like a struggle to keep up with, and a partner that is feeling neglected, all the while her own body is screaming at her with different ailments and challenges. I had a patient whose elderly parents had dementia and neurodegenerative conditions that drastically changed their quality of life along with hers. She was instantly swept into the role of a caretaker for her parents. This role reversal that many women deal with comes with many layers of emotions, challenges, and even gifts. Seeing one's parents change and lose the identity of someone you could turn to for support carries with it triggers from not just this moment but the stories of your childhood. There is a cultural, societal, and self-imposed expectation to try to do everything you can to support them by sacrificing your own health. I've seen this in my own family and in so many of my patients. This pull in multiple directions creates so much guilt and shame that these women begin to lose themselves in the process. Wanting to do the best they can and not knowing where or how to draw the boundaries necessary to take care of themselves in the process.

To create healthy boundaries, a woman needs to be able to use her voice. She needs to be able to communicate with confidence and a level of assertiveness so her message is clear and kind. However, most of us women weren't always given room to find that confident voice. Nor was it modeled by the women around us. Whether at home, at work, or in the doctor's office, many women find it hard to fully share their feelings and what they need. This loss of voice or this inability to express keeps her emotions hidden and stuck in her body. When a woman feels unheard, it can create frustration and anger that has nowhere to go.

One organ that often gets the brunt of this inability to speak her truth is the thyroid. Research has shown that repressed anger can increase cortisol in your body due to the fight-or-flight state, and this cortisol decreases thyroid hormone production and conversion of T4 (thyroxine) to the active thyroid hormone T3 (triiodothyronine), lowering your energy, increasing your susceptibility to autoimmune disease of the thyroid, inflammation, and depression.

The thyroid's hormones play a huge role in your reproductive health. It oversees the energy production of every cell in your body. Without it, the communication between brain and body are compromised, leaving the cells in a state of starvation. There are various stressors that can impact the thyroid. It is the largest endocrine organ and especially vulnerable to chemical and emotional stressors. Chemical stressors like heavy metals—specifically, mercury, lead, and cadmium present in everyday products and food—seem to create the most harm toward the thyroid. They block receptor sites in the thyroid and diminish its ability to function and communicate.

For example, lead and cadmium are found in pesticides that are sprayed on fruits and vegetables, and they both impact thyroid function. Lead specifically tends to decrease levels of TSH and upregulate thyroid peroxidase antibodies, causing an autoimmune condition of the thyroid, while cadmium binds to receptors upregulating thyroglobulin antibodies and is also a major disruptor of estrogen function. Emotional stressors also take their toll on this organ.

Many women who have experienced trauma—whether in the past or in their present struggles to be heard—often face challenges with their thyroid health. I've worked with women dealing with conditions ranging from thyroid nodules and cysts to autoimmune thyroid disease and

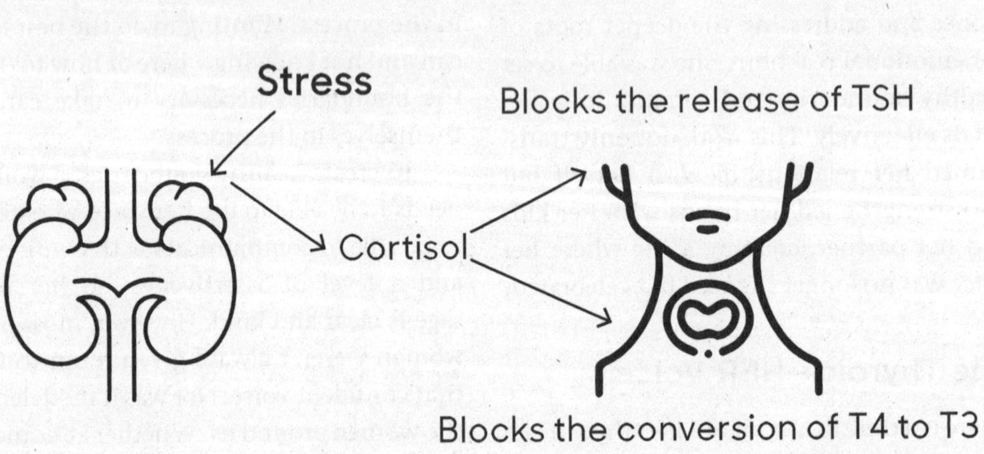

| EFFECTS OF HIGH THYROID HORMONES | EFFECTS OF LOW THYROID HORMONES |
|---|---|
| Sweating | Weight gain |
| Anxiety | Hair loss |
| Insomnia | Depression |
| Weight loss | Dry skin |
| Irritability | Cold extremities |

even thyroid cancer. Every one of them carried a story of trauma. One woman lived with the memory of an abusive father who committed suicide in front of her. Another endured the pain of being raped by a stranger, while yet another faced that same violation at the hands of someone she knew. One was the youngest in her family, constantly fighting to be seen and heard, while another lived a life dictated by her parents' expectations, leaving no room for her own dreams.

In all these stories, a common thread emerged: the experience of their power being taken away and their voices silenced. And while we may not all have experienced traumas of this magnitude, many of us can recall moments when we wished we had spoken up, had the confidence to express our truth, or truly believed that our voice mattered.

The silence imposed by these moments—whether by others or ourselves—has a profound impact on our health. Your ability to express yourself influences your physical, mental, and emotional well-being in ways you may not even realize. While it may feel like you've lost the power to choose in these moments, reclaiming your voice is always possible. Even in the aftermath of silence, the choice to speak up and heal remains within your grasp.

By fully expressing your needs, you can clear frustration, release anger, and transform sadness into a feeling of capability, strength, resilience, and confidence. The more you speak up, the more you ask for what you need, the more trust you build within yourself, the easier it gets to use your voice.

We sometimes think we need to sacrifice our voice to keep the peace, but what if we have it all wrong? What if speaking up creates an opportunity toward healing for all parties involved? What if we can say to our aging parents struggling with their health that you want to show up as your best self but can't when you are feeling overworked and overwhelmed? What if that opens conversations on how everyone can work together to support each other? What if when you went into your doctor's appointment, you went in with the intention that no matter the response from the other side, "I am going to share my story and ask for what I want because this is my health and my life"? What if that perpetrator that took your voice away could no longer have power over you and your voice? What if you speak what happened to you to release that hold and to forgive yourself? I know it isn't as easy as it sounds, as there are layers to your why, and at the same time, you can make a choice today to be brave, one experience at a time.

## DHEA—HER Vitality

Dehydroepiandrosterone (DHEA) is one of the most crucial yet overlooked hormones when it comes to women's reproductive health, especially dehydroepiandrosterone sulphate (DHEA-S), which is shown to fluctuate in your luteal phase—starting to decrease in the early luteal phase, low in midluteal, and it begins to rise again in late luteal. Produced primarily by the adrenal glands, DHEA serves as a precursor to both estrogen and testosterone, making it essential for fertility, libido, bone density, mood stability, cardiovascular health, recovery, and even cognitive function. When DHEA levels are optimal, women often feel vibrant, energetic, and emotionally resilient. However, chronic stress and unresolved trauma can deplete DHEA levels, throwing the entire hormonal ecosystem into disarray.

I once had a patient, Sophie, a 38-year-old woman who came to me feeling completely exhausted. She had been trying to conceive for two years with no success. Her cycles were irregular, her libido was nonexistent, and she struggled with brain fog that made even simple daily tasks feel overwhelming. When we tested her hormones, her DHEA levels were significantly low. As we dug deeper into her story, it became clear that years of chronic stress—balancing a demanding job, caregiving for a sick parent, and suppressing the emotional wounds from a past abusive relationship—had drained her adrenal reserves. Her body had been prioritizing survival over reproduction, shutting down the very pathways that supported hormonal balance.

DHEA is often called the "youth hormone" because of its role in vitality, but more than that, it acts as a protective buffer against the physiological damage of long-term stress. When stress is unrelenting, the

| EFFECTS OF HIGH DHEA | EFFECTS OF LOW DHEA |
|---|---|
| Irregular cycles | Fatigue |
| Hirsutism | Depression |
| Hair loss | Low libido |
| Infertility | Joint pain |
| Oily skin | Anxiety |
| Low libido | Increased risk of cardiovascular disease |
| Acne | Increased risk of osteoporosis |
| Anxiety | Impaired immune health |
| PCOS | Brain fog |

body redirects its resources to produce cortisol, the survival hormone, at the expense of DHEA. Over time, this depletion not only affects fertility but also accelerates aging, weakens immunity, and contributes to mood disorders. For Sophie, the solution wasn't just about supplementing DHEA; it was about addressing the emotional weight she had been carrying for years. Through adrenal support, nervous system regulation, and deep emotional healing, her body slowly began to shift out of survival mode. Within a few months, her cycles became regular, her energy returned, and not long after, she conceived naturally.

Sophie's story is a reminder that hormones don't exist in isolation. DHEA isn't just a number on a lab test—it's a reflection of how safe, nourished, and supported your body feels. If you've been feeling depleted, disconnected, or like your reproductive health is slipping away, it may be time to look beyond just your hormones and into the deeper layers of stress, trauma, and self-care that shape your well-being. Healing isn't just about boosting levels—it's about restoring balance from the inside out and finding clarity in what you need and the vitality in your body.

CHAPTER 5

# The Root of Your Reactions

We all experience moments when our reactions feel bigger than the situation in front of us—whether it's anxiety, sadness, irritability, or rage. These emotional waves often feel automatic, but they're not random. They are rooted in a deeper internal landscape: your hormones, your emotional patterns, and the unspoken stories that live inside you.

Think about the last time you were in a tense moment with a partner, child, or friend. Were you fully present? Or were you caught in your own internal swirl—feeling overwhelmed by emotion, bracing for judgment, or replaying old fears or hurts? Often, our reactions are not just about what's happening now, but about what our body remembers, what our hormones are signaling, and what our past has taught us to expect.

This is where the heart becomes your guide. When you pause and connect with your heart, you open a doorway to deeper listening—not just to others, but to yourself. You begin to ask important questions: *What am I feeling? Why am I feeling this way? Is this my truth, my fear, or my hormones speaking?*

In many traditions, the heart is seen as a source of wisdom. In Sufi mysticism, it holds your divine spark and inner knowing. In Chinese medicine, the heart is the seat of love, compassion, and forgiveness—the place where healing begins. Yet in our everyday lives, it's easy to lose touch with that wisdom. Pain, betrayal, and stress can cause us to armor up, believing protection comes through shutting down. But your heart's wisdom never disappears—it waits patiently to be remembered.

Think back to the first rhythm you ever knew: your mother's heartbeat. That steady drumbeat wrapped you in safety, long before you had language to understand what you were feeling. You knew, instinctively, that you were held. That you were enough.

Over time, life pulls us away from that truth. Experiences shape us, hormones shift us, and expectations weigh us down. We begin to forget how to trust ourselves, how to stay connected to our emotional center. But your heart remains your anchor. Every emotion—grief, joy, fear, anger—is a messenger guiding you back to yourself.

In this chapter, you'll explore how different emotions are shaped by your hormonal landscape—alongside reflective questions, supportive practices, and tools to help you better understand your personal relationship with each one.

As we explore hormonal anxiety, depression, and emotional reactivity in the pages ahead, I invite you to approach these experiences with compassion and curiosity. You are not broken—you are responding. And within those responses lies the invitation to understand your body, your hormones, and your truth more deeply.

## Your Body Expresses Your Emotions

When you see a child lost in her joy, curiosity, and wonder, it's hard to imagine that one day, she might experience pain or carry invisible wounds. Yet, life has a way of shaping us—micro and even macro traumas leave their marks, changing how we see ourselves and how we connect with the world. Looking at that child, we can't know the stories her nervous system is recording, the neuronal pathways being wired by her experiences at home, school, or even on the playground.

The truth is, we've all had moments that altered how we express ourselves. Moments that planted seeds of shame, made us question our worth, and dimmed our light. Maybe it was being excluded on the playground, feeling like your sibling was loved differently, sensing discomfort around a certain relative, or a deeply painful experience of violated boundaries. In each of these moments, a piece of your power, innocence, or joy was overshadowed.

These experiences often get buried in our subconscious, and without realizing it, we form invisible contracts with ourselves to stay safe. You might become someone who always needs to be in control, someone who strives to please others, or someone who blends into any environment to feel like you belong. These protective patterns are reinforced by your emotional system, hormones, and neurotransmitters working together to create a safety response.

Over time, triggers—like a smell, a tone of voice, or even a familiar feeling—can awaken those old survival stories. The emotional brain sends signals to the hormonal system, preparing you to react and protect yourself in ways you might not even understand. But here's the hope: With reflection and intention, you can begin to unravel these old circuits. You can build new pathways, ones rooted in safety, trust, and connection.

There are key moments in life when we start to notice changes within ourselves. We begin to see layers of emotions we've buried and shades of experience we didn't realize were there. These moments often bring physical and emotional discomfort, especially tied to hormonal shifts. In Chinese medicine, the reproductive organs are thought to hold on to unresolved stories from the past. When we cling to these stories—carrying old pain and unresolved emotions—they can energetically settle in these organs, leading to the discomforts we feel in our bodies every day.

The connection between trauma, emotions, and hormones is becoming better understood as shown by a recent study stating, "Cumulatively, much of the current literature suggests that the link between reproductive and emotional health instigated by trauma may have severe consequences for a woman's wellbeing throughout every life stage." Trauma can take many forms—neglect, household dysfunction, racial stress, sexual assault, physical or emotional abuse. It includes any experience that forced you to abandon or redefine yourself to feel safe, creating a constant cycle of stress between your hormones and emotions.

I once heard trauma categorized into two types: abandonment and invasion. If you reflect on the moments that have left lasting imprints, you may find they fit into one of these categories. By identifying and addressing these core wounds, we can begin to heal the many instances where our power was taken away.

## UNDERSTANDING YOUR WOUNDS: A SELF-REFLECTION AND BODY AWARENESS QUESTIONNAIRE

These wounds don't just live in your mind—they live in your body. Your nervous system, hormones, and emotional responses are shaped by these past experiences, influencing everything from your energy levels to your physical health and relationships.

This questionnaire will help you identify the root of your wounds, understand how they manifest in your body, and bring awareness to areas that may need healing.

Take your time, find a quiet space, and reflect with honesty and compassion.

### Section 1: Identifying Invasion Wounds

(These wounds often stem from feeling overpowered, violated, or controlled—either physically, emotionally, or mentally.)

- Did you ever feel like you had to shrink yourself, silence your voice, or comply with someone else's expectations to feel safe?
- Were your emotional, physical, or energetic boundaries ever ignored or disrespected?
- Did you grow up in an environment where control or punishment was used as a means of discipline?
- Do you feel hypervigilant, like you must always be "on guard" in certain relationships or situations?

- Are you uncomfortable with physical closeness, touch, or intimacy, even in safe relationships?
- Do you struggle with trusting others, always waiting for something to go wrong?
- Do you find yourself overexplaining, overapologizing, or justifying your needs out of fear of someone's reaction?
- Does confrontation or conflict trigger a deep sense of fear or helplessness?
- Have you ever felt like your body doesn't fully belong to you, as if you've detached from it to survive?
- When setting boundaries, do you experience guilt or fear that you will be punished, rejected, or hurt?

Where do you feel this in your body?

- Do you clench your jaw when feeling controlled or overwhelmed?
- Do you carry tension in your shoulders as if holding the weight of the world?
- Do you experience chest tightness or shallow breathing when feeling unsafe?
- Does your stomach tighten or ache when recalling boundary violations?
- Do you feel numbness or detachment from parts of your body?

---

## Section 2: Identifying Abandonment Wounds

(These wounds often come from feeling emotionally neglected, dismissed, or left unsupported—physically or emotionally.)

- Did you grow up feeling like you had to take care of others emotionally or physically because no one was taking care of you?
- Were you often left alone—either physically, emotionally, or both—when you needed comfort or guidance?
- Did you feel like your emotions were dismissed, ignored, or shamed? ("Stop crying," "Get over it," "You're too sensitive.")
- Did you fear that love, affection, or approval were conditional—that you had to earn them?
- Do you find yourself clinging to relationships, even if they aren't healthy, out of fear of being alone?

- Do you feel like you need to prove your worth through productivity, perfection, or caretaking?
- Do you struggle with self-trust, always looking to others for validation or reassurance?
- Do you have difficulty expressing your needs, fearing they will be rejected or seen as too much?
- Does loneliness feel overwhelming, even when you are surrounded by people?
- Do you notice patterns of attracting emotionally unavailable people or those who make you feel like you must chase love?
- Where do you feel this in your body?
- Do you experience tightness in your throat, as if words are stuck inside you?
- Do you feel a hollow or aching sensation in your chest when you fear rejection?
- Do you hold tension in your hips, as if bracing yourself for loss?
- Do you experience low energy or fatigue from constantly giving to others?
- Do you get frequent digestive issues or stomach knots when feeling unsupported?

---

## Section 3: Reflection and Integration

- Which section resonated more deeply with you—Invasion, Abandonment, or both?
- How do these wounds show up in your daily life, relationships, and self-perception?
- What coping mechanisms have you used to navigate these wounds (perfectionism, overworking, emotional eating, avoidance, people-pleasing, etc.)?
- What do you need to feel safe in your body and in your relationships today?
- If you could speak to your younger self, the one who first experienced this wound, what would you tell her?

Awareness is the first step toward healing. This exercise isn't meant to dwell in the pain, but rather to bring clarity to the patterns that have shaped your emotional and physical and hormonal health—and to remind you that healing is possible.

Your body has been holding on to these wounds, but it is also capable of letting go, healing, and rewriting the story. Take a deep breath, offer yourself kindness, and know that you are not alone in this journey.

Over time, we've all found ways to hide the parts of ourselves that feel fragile, hurt, or in need of help. But when we rebuild the relationship with ourselves by understanding ourselves, we create space to express who we truly are. This allows us to approach relationships from a place of safety and inner strength, rather than hiding our vulnerabilities. When you start to heal your heart and show compassion to yourself, you open the door to having compassion for others. The healing begins with you; the healing begins with your heart and understanding of yourself and the why behind the emotions you carry and feel.

## Hormonal Anxiety and Worry

In Taoism, anxiety and worry are described as "hooking of the heart," a form of holding on. In Buddhism, they are considered the root of suffering, while in Sikhism, anxiety is seen as the opposite of faith, arising when we focus more on the future than the present moment. Across ancient and modern traditions, anxiety has been recognized as a fundamental part of the human experience.

If humanity has been dealing with anxiety for so long—and we now understand so much about the nervous system—why do we still struggle with it? Why does this cycle of worry and suffering persist? Perhaps it's because we haven't taken the time to truly understand it—where it comes from, what lessons it holds, and how it can create challenges when left unchecked.

Anxiety pulls us out of the present moment and into an imagined future, often filled with worst-case scenarios. While a little anxiety can be healthy—helping us stay alert and make thoughtful decisions—it's often a protective response after trauma, a way for the brain to shield us from similar pain. Interestingly, anxiety and excitement share similar physiological responses—an accelerated heart rate, increased energy, and a heightened sense of alertness. Both emotions prepare the body for action, but the difference lies in how we interpret them. Anxiety often carries a sense of dread or fear of what could go wrong, while excitement feels like anticipation of something positive. In this way, they're two sides of the same coin. Without experiencing the tension and restlessness that anxiety brings, we might struggle to fully savor the peace and calm of contentment. The contrast between these states allows us to appreciate moments of stillness, joy, and ease, making them all the more meaningful. Anxiety, when understood and reframed, can remind us of what we value and help us cultivate gratitude for the times when life feels lighter and more balanced.

According to the Anxiety and Depression Association of America, women between puberty and age 50 are twice as likely to experience anxiety as men. Why? The answer lies in the way our shifting hormones affect the brain and shape our perceptions. These changing perceptions can alter our emotional states, influence our actions, and even impact our relationships—especially when we don't understand why we feel the way we do.

As we discussed in Chapter 3, a woman's brain is wired to anticipate fear and pain more than a man's, making it harder to suppress feelings of fear in daily situations that may remind her of past trauma or moments when she felt unsafe. Anxiety acts like a warning alarm, keeping her on high alert and ready to fight, flee, or freeze.

In today's world, many of us feel like we're under constant stress, with our sense of safety always in question. This makes it difficult to shift from anxiety into calm, leaving us more reactive and overwhelmed, especially with our kids, partners, or anyone who crosses our path.

During puberty, when hormones are trying to find their rhythm, girls are especially vulnerable to anxiety. It's not just the internal chemical shifts; it's also the discomfort and unfamiliarity of their changing bodies. This same vulnerability follows women throughout their reproductive years, from pregnancy to childbirth, through perimenopause, and finally into menopause, as their bodies and hormones continue to change.

## The Root of Hormonal Anxiety

Anxiety can be influenced by many factors—learned behaviors, hormonal changes, or even stress experienced in the womb. When a pregnant woman feels high levels of stress and anxiety, it can impact her baby's HPA axis, making the child more prone to higher cortisol levels and reactivity later in life.

For example, a study of 496 mothers in Mexico City measured their cortisol levels and compared them to their children's anxiety scores at ages 8 through 11. The results showed that mothers who experienced higher cortisol and anxiety during pregnancy had children with higher anxiety levels as preteens. This gives us insight into how our own state today affects us and our families.

When life feels overwhelming—whether it's rushing to get the kids out the door, meeting a work deadline, or feeling unsupported by your partner—these everyday stressors can heighten anxiety, especially during times of hormonal changes. Women are most vulnerable to this during two key phases of life: puberty and perimenopause.

We often talk about teen mood swings, but the emotional impact of perimenopause is just now being recognized. As estrogen declines, so does your ability to shift out of fear. Estrogen helps calm the fear response, which is why women feel more confident during the first half of their cycle. But as estrogen levels drop—either in the week before your period or during perimenopause—you may feel more anxious, sensitive, and out of control.

This hormonal shift also increases sensitivity to your environment, a phenomenon called psychosocial sensitivity. For example, you might feel stressed before attending an event or anxious about the energy it will take to be there. Estrogen and serotonin, which work together to help you feel calm and process sounds, both decline. That's why your kids' once-adorable voices might suddenly feel like nails on a chalkboard or why little noises, like your husband's chewing, feel unbearable—leading to even more anxiety.

When we talk about anxiety in women, it's important to understand that it doesn't appear out of nowhere—it follows a trajectory shaped by both biology and lived experience. From childhood through menopause, a woman's hormonal landscape, life transitions, and social conditioning all play a role in how anxiety is experienced and expressed.

In **childhood**, anxiety levels between boys and girls are relatively similar. But early influences—such as trauma, neglect, poor nutrition, family dynamics, and environmental stress—can begin to shape the nervous system and lay the groundwork for future emotional sensitivity.

As a girl enters **puberty**, hormonal fluctuations in estrogen and progesterone introduce new emotional and physiological vulnerabilities. Changes in brain development, increasing social stressors, body image pressures, and even early use of hormonal birth control can all contribute to heightened anxiety during this stage.

In **adulthood**, hormonal shifts continue to play a role, especially for women who experience premenstrual anxiety (PMA) or PMDD. These biological sensitivities often collide with cultural and career expectations, alcohol use, time stress, and the ongoing pressure to "do it all," creating the perfect storm for chronic anxiety.

During **motherhood**, anxiety can intensify due to a sharp drop in reproductive hormones following childbirth. Added to this are the emotional demands of a major identity shift, sleep deprivation, lack of support systems, and the constant juggling of responsibilities—all of which can leave women feeling overwhelmed and emotionally fragile.

As women move into **perimenopause**, anxiety may resurface or intensify, this time driven by unpredictable hormone fluctuations. This phase is often called "reverse puberty," where mood swings, irritability, and emotional instability can feel overwhelming, especially as the hormonal protection of earlier years begins to fade.

Finally, in **menopause and postmenopause**, consistently low levels of estrogen and other key hormones can impact mood regulation, cognitive clarity, and emotional resilience. These physical changes are often compounded by deeper existential stressors, such as shifting identities, changing relationships, societal invisibility, and a growing awareness of aging and mortality.

Understanding this trajectory helps us view anxiety not as a personal failure or flaw, but as a natural response to complex hormonal, emotional, and social dynamics throughout a woman's life.

When left unrecognized, this one state can change how you show up in all your relationships, at work, and in new opportunities. The impact it holds is profound, but the healing that comes from understanding it is equally transformative. Unlearning the pattern of anxiety takes conscious work, but this work cannot be complete without understanding how your hormones play a role in it.

In the previous chapter, you learned how progesterone affects anxiety and how most women are depleted due to excess estrogen from environmental sources like pesticides, beauty products, plastics, and chronic stress. This constant stress causes the body to convert progesterone into cortisol, robbing the brain of progesterone's calming effects.

It's reported that 80 percent of women in their reproductive years experience mood changes, particularly anxiety, during the luteal phase of their cycle. This is when progesterone should be at its highest, helping you feel calm. Beyond hormonal changes, many women have come to identify with being anxious—it feels so familiar that they believe they need anxiety to stay productive and get through the day. But it's time to change that.

Anxiety doesn't have to be negative. Instead, it can be a signal to get curious about what it's trying to teach you. Most often, it's trying to keep you safe from emotional or physical harm. However, when overused, anxiety disconnects us from the present by pulling us into future worries. The opposite of this state is mindfulness—being fully present, feeling content, and knowing you're enough as you are.

I've personally noticed that when I'm stuck projecting fears or expectations about the future, I miss out on the gifts of the present moment, like time with my boys. When life feels like it's moving too fast, it's often because we're stuck in a mindset of "not enough"—always reaching for the next thing. Ironically, the same anxiety about not having enough time is what makes us feel that way in the first place.

When we understand this, we can shift our perspective, create space for presence, and make anxiety work for us instead of against us. By embracing the moment, we can stretch time and feel more grounded in the here and now.

## GUIDED MEDITATION: MEETING YOUR HORMONAL ANXIETY

Find a quiet, comfortable space where you won't be disturbed. Sit or lie down, close your eyes, and take a deep breath in through your nose . . . hold it for a moment . . . and exhale slowly through your mouth with a deep sigh. Let your breath become your anchor, guiding you into a place of deep connection and curiosity with yourself.

### Step 1: Inviting Your Anxiety to Appear

Imagine yourself standing in a peaceful, open field. The air is warm, the sky is soft, and the ground beneath you feels steady and supportive. In the distance, you see a figure approaching. This is your anxiety—not as an enemy, not as something to fear, but as a part of you that has been working hard to protect you.

As the figure comes closer, take a moment to observe it. What does it look like? How does it carry itself? What is its energy like? Maybe it appears as a wise old woman, a cautious child, or even a fierce protector standing guard. However it looks, know that this is a part of you that has been trying to keep you safe.

### Step 2: Giving It a Name

Gently ask this part of you, "What is your name?" Listen for the first name or word that comes to mind. Maybe it's *Doubt*, *Overwhelm*, *the Watcher*, or something entirely unique to you. Whatever it is, accept it without judgment.

Now greet it and let it know, "I see you and I can feel you. I know you've been here for a long time and have been working hard to protect me."

### Step 3: Understanding Its Purpose

With curiosity, ask:

- "What are you trying to protect me from?"
- "What lesson are you trying to teach me?"
- "Why do you show up in these moments?"

Allow the answers to arise naturally. Maybe your anxiety has been trying to shield you from failure, rejection, or past wounds. Maybe it has been carrying the weight of expectations placed upon you, or maybe it simply wants you to slow down and listen.

If it feels resistant or unclear, that's okay. You can gently reassure it: "I appreciate you looking out for me, but I want to understand you better. You don't have to fight me—I am listening."

---

### Step 4: Rewriting the Relationship

Now imagine extending your hand to this part of you. Feel a sense of warmth and compassion as you say:

- "You don't have to work so hard anymore. I hear you, and I will honor your wisdom."
- "I am safe. I am supported. I am learning to trust myself."
- "We can walk together, but I get to choose how I respond."

As you say these words, notice if the figure begins to soften. Maybe it nods in understanding, maybe it places a hand on your shoulder, or maybe it simply steps back, trusting you to lead.

---

### Step 5: Integrating Peace

Now visualize this figure merging gently into your heart, no longer separate from you, but a part of your wisdom. Take a deep breath in, and as you exhale, feel a newfound sense of ease spreading through your body. Your hormones, your mind, your emotions—they are all connected, and you have the power to guide them with love, not fear.

When you're ready, slowly bring awareness back to your surroundings. Wiggle your fingers and toes, and when you open your eyes, carry this newfound understanding with you. Anxiety is not your enemy—it is a messenger. And now you know how to listen.

**YOUR AFFIRMATION:**

*I am in control of my body, my emotions, and my thoughts.*
*I listen with compassion, and I move forward with trust.*

## Hormonal Depression and Grief

According to the *Diagnostic and Statistical Manual of Mental Disorders (DSM-5)*, published by the American Psychiatric Association, the following are signs and symptoms of clinical depression:

- Feelings of sadness, emptiness or hopelessness
- Angry outbursts, irritability or frustration, even over small matters
- Loss of interest or pleasure in most or all normal activities, such as sex, hobbies, or sports
- Sleep disturbances, including insomnia or sleeping too much
- Tiredness and lack of energy, so even small tasks take extra effort
- Reduced appetite and weight loss or increased cravings for food and weight gain
- Anxiety, agitation, or restlessness
- Slowed thinking, speaking, or body movements
- Feelings of worthlessness or guilt, fixating on past failures or self-blame
- Trouble thinking, concentrating, making decisions, and remembering things
- Frequent or recurrent thoughts about death, suicidal thoughts, suicide attempts
- Unexplained physical problems, such as back pain or headaches

These symptoms can also indicate hormonal imbalances, so how can we tell the difference between clinical depression and hormone-related depression? Hormonal depression often comes in waves during times of hormonal shifts, like puberty, premenstruation, postpartum, perimenopause, or menopause. When hormones like estrogen or testosterone drop, neurotransmitters like serotonin and dopamine also decrease, directly impacting your mood and how you process the world around you.

For example, women with PMS, particularly premenstrual depression (PMS-D), may feel low and fatigued in the weeks leading up to their period due to reduced serotonin levels or even an underactive thyroid. A more severe form of PMS-D is premenstrual dysphoric disorder (PMDD), where mood shifts become overwhelming and debilitating.

One key reason for these emotional shifts is unresolved past trauma. An Australian descriptive study found that 83 percent of women with PMDD had a history of early childhood abuse, with emotional abuse being the most common. Often, the deep emotional reactions we feel in the present stem from an inner child still seeking the care and nurturing she missed growing up. When hormones drop—whether it's in the last week of your cycle, after pregnancy, or during perimenopause—the protective "veil" that kept past traumas buried is lifted. Without that hormonal buffer, your brain may respond with depression as it processes feelings of loss, diminished self-worth, and a shaken sense of identity.

Not all women with hormonal depression have experienced abuse. However, any level of stress can affect your body's nutrient levels and disrupt your digestion. This makes it harder to absorb nutrients and support the microbiome—the community of microbes in your body that helps break down food, produce energy, vitamins, and neurotransmitters like serotonin, and defend against illness. Under stress, we often make choices that drain our body and brain instead of nourishing them. We may eat more processed, sugary foods, skip exercise, or stay up later than we should. These daily habits affect the nutrients our body stores, produces, and uses. Low levels of amino acids like tyrosine, vitamins like $B_6$, and minerals like zinc can disrupt hormone balance, making it harder for your brain and gut to produce the right neurochemical mix for joy and happiness.

Depression, I find, has layers to it just like any other emotion. When experiencing this state, it is easy to look at all the things that are not working in your life rather than seeing the gifts it has to offer right now. Those wrapped in this sadness are often still stuck in past stories and have a hard time moving into the present. When working with these emotions and the hormonal picture that contributes to them, I make sure to address the past hurts and patterns that are not allowing a woman to see her life from the lens of the present and from the lens of hope. Your past can inform your present but doesn't have to define it. How freeing is that?

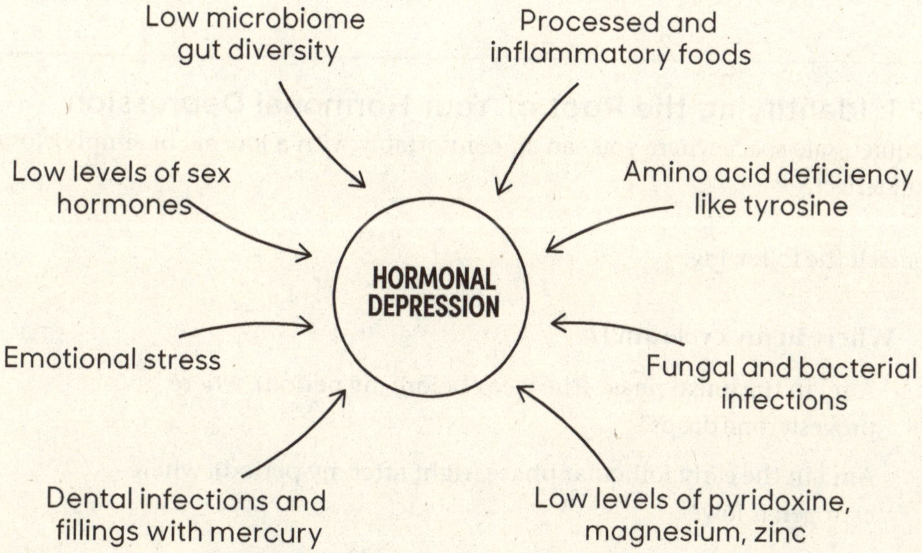

I know depression isn't a switch you can turn on and off, and I know by changing perspective, by supporting the body and brain, by choosing a mindset that helps you look toward hope, you can exponentially change how your brain is processing your life and your relationships so you can feel the joy that is your birthright. As I mentioned in an earlier chapter, sadness at its root is connected to a sense of satisfaction. Depression may also be that reminder of the fullness and richness of the past and the satisfaction one had felt and may now be missing in the present. Depression may also be a guide for us to understand our wounds and the beliefs we have carried because of them.

Each woman's medicine to understand and transform this state is going to be unique to her. Dancing has been a gift in my life that has pulled me out of this state countless times. The following is a way you can identify what you need to help shift your state during the heavy times.

---

## EXERCISE FOR IDENTIFYING THE ROOT OF HORMONAL DEPRESSION & SHIFTING YOUR STATE

Hormonal depression can feel like a heavy fog—one that blurs your thoughts, dampens your energy, and makes everything feel overwhelming. When you find yourself in this state, instead of resisting it, try sitting with it. Your body is communicating something important. This exercise will help you tune in, identify the root cause, and shift your emotional and physical state using breath, movement, and visualization.

---

### STEP 1: Identifying the Root of Your Hormonal Depression

Find a quiet, safe space where you can sit comfortably with a journal or simply close your eyes and reflect.

Ask yourself the following:

1. **Where in my cycle am I?**
    - Am I in the luteal phase (the week before my period), where progesterone drops?
    - Am I in the early follicular phase (right after my period), where estrogen is low?
    - Am I in perimenopause or postmenopausal?

- Have I had any major changes or transitions in my life?
- Have I been skipping meals, not sleeping enough, or under stress, which could be affecting my blood sugar and hormones?

2. **What emotion is most dominant right now?**
*(circle or name what resonates)*

- **Sadness:** Am I grieving something (a past version of me, a relationship, an unmet expectation)?
- **Frustration:** Is something in my life not aligning with what I need?
- **Loneliness:** Have I been withdrawing from connection or not feeling seen?
- **Guilt/Shame:** Am I being too hard on myself or replaying past mistakes?
- **Exhaustion:** Have I been overextending myself without rest?

3. **Where do I feel this in my body?**
*(place your hand there as you reflect)*

- **Heart/Chest:** Emotional grief, heartbreak, lack of self-love
- **Throat:** Repressed emotions, unspoken needs
- **Stomach/Womb:** Intuition being ignored, fear of uncertainty
- **Neck/Shoulders:** Carrying too many responsibilities, feeling unsupported

4. **If my depression had a voice, what would it say?**

- "I need rest."
- "I feel unsafe."
- "I am carrying too much."
- "I feel alone."
- "I need to release control."

Journal any thoughts or words that surface. The simple act of identifying your hormonal state and naming your emotions will bring clarity and empowerment.

## STEP 2: Shifting Your State—Breath, Movement & Meditation

Once you've acknowledged the root cause, your body needs a somatic (physical) shift to release the emotional weight and recalibrate your nervous system.

### Option 1: Breathwork—The Hormonal Reset Breath

*(This technique helps activate your parasympathetic nervous system, calming the hormonal storm in your body.)*

- **Step 1:** Take a deep inhale through your nose for 4 counts, hold at the top for 4 counts.
- **Step 2:** Exhale through your mouth with a sighing sound for 6 counts.
- **Step 3:** Repeat for 5 minutes, imagining all stagnant energy melting away with each exhale.

*For deeper release:* On the last exhale, **stick out your tongue (Lion's Breath)** and let out any frustration or sadness.

### Option 2: Movement—Shake & Flow

*(This one I love! This practice releases tension and stored trauma from the nervous system, creating immediate relief.)*

- **Step 1:** Stand with feet hip width apart and gently shake your body (start with your hands, then arms, shoulders, legs, and head—like you're shaking off the heaviness).
- **Step 2:** Set a timer for 2 minutes and play upbeat music (drumming, tribal beats, or any song that makes you feel powerful).
- **Step 3:** Close your eyes and move however your body wants—sway, bounce, or dance.
- **Step 4:** End with Child's Pose or lying flat on the floor, hands on belly, breathing deeply.

*Notice how your energy shifts after—your body is releasing and recalibrating!*

### Option 3: Visualization Meditation—Meeting Your Hormonal Self

*Find a quiet space, close your eyes, and take a deep breath.*

Imagine stepping into a sacred, peaceful place—a garden, the ocean, a warm forest.

Allow yourself to feel the fullness of the moments and all the sensations connected to it. The smell of the flowers, feeling the mist from the sea, or hearing the birds. Allow each sense to experience the presence in that sacred and safe space. In front of you, you notice a strong presence of familiarity and warmth. As you open your eyes, you see that in front of you stands a gentle, powerful version of yourself, holding a light in her hands.

She whispers: "I have been waiting for you." She takes your hand and asks you to sit across from her, giving you permission to ask her anything.

- What do I need to learn from this feeling right now?
- What is my body trying to tell me?
- What can I, and what do I, need to let go of today to release the weight I carry?

As you ask the questions, you see visions of your past. Moments that have been imprinted into your body and moments that you have been carrying on your back. Without a word she hands you the light—symbolizing wisdom, healing, and clarity. Instinctively you begin to blow into the light and notice the visions moving into the light, leaving you feeling lighter and lighter as each vision and the tight hold it had on your body gets released. She takes the light from you, embracing you and whispering in your ear: "You are safe, you are worthy, and you are so much more than those moments, you are simply enough."

**Take three deep breaths and return to the present moment.**

## Grief as a Reminder of Self-Love

A common conversation I have with my patients navigating major life transitions—whether preparing for motherhood, adjusting to life with a new baby, or entering perimenopause and embracing a new phase—is about their experience of grief. This grief often brings a deep sadness that might be mistaken for depression but is, in reality, a natural response to where they are in their hormonal and life journey.

I find grief is a beautiful emotion that reminds us of the love we have for life and the relations we get to experience in it, especially the relation to ourselves. When a young woman is grieving her childhood innocence once she starts to bleed, she is also celebrating stepping to womanhood and into her own power. When a new mother is grieving her old body, she is also celebrating the body that carried life inside of it. When a woman is starting her journey to say goodbye to her reproductive years, she is also celebrating who she was and who she gets to become.

Grief and sadness are gifts. They give us permission to step into the shadows of ourselves, into the darkness and into a space of deep reflection, giving us an opportunity to use our own light for clarity toward what is next. This darkness gives us permission to go deep into our caves to reflect and reconnect. To feel and to release. Grief and sadness are an opportunity to cleanse and let go. Just like our monthly cycle.

As the lining of your uterus sheds, you not only release physically but also have an opportunity to release emotionally. Each month, a part of your story can fade away, creating space for something new to emerge. During your period, if you're in sync with the moon, you might bleed during the new moon—a time of darkness and introspection, inviting you to turn inward. The new moon is a powerful time for introspection and renewal, mirroring the natural phases women experience during their cycles. Just as the moon wanes into darkness, this phase invites us to pause, reflect, and turn inward. The new moon represents a blank canvas—a moment of stillness before new energy and intentions emerge. For women, this can be a deeply sacred time to connect with their inner selves, shed old emotions, and plant seeds for personal growth.

Many women describe feeling like a completely different person as their period begins or ends, as though they've let go of the emotions weighing them down. They often feel lighter, more content, and ready to embrace hope and joy in their daily lives. However, if the physical body isn't supported during the hormonal shifts leading into the next phase, women can get stuck in a cycle of monthly discomfort.

This cycle not only affects women but also impacts their families, who may struggle to understand or provide the support needed for the emotional and physical changes that occur throughout the month.

There was a young patient once. On the outside she was this beautiful, vibrant, loving, smart, and hardworking woman that many would say had it all together. However, if you knew her inner world or if you could hear her inner world, you would hear the loudest inner critic. A voice so loud that it once told her to carve the words "I hate life" on her arm, that is pain she was hiding inside of her. She was wanting to take her own life because she felt so worthless and trapped in self-hate.

They say how you speak to your children becomes your inner voice, and hearing things like "you make me sick" from her parents imprinted in her psyche that she was the cause of suffering for the people she loved. Never really feeling like anything she did was enough and never really feeling like she could be happy or even deserved to be happy. Depression and sadness became her friends. She learned to mask it, suppress it, and keep it all to herself, until of course her body had enough.

Her bleeds were so heavy that she would have to take days off school. Her uterus was inflamed, she had cancerous cells on her cervix, and she knew that the sadness and loneliness she felt even when surrounded by family and friends was her body's way of speaking to her because something needed to change. She also had PCOS, and studies have shown us that women with PCOS tend to have higher amounts of cortisol and low amounts of serotonin, making them more susceptible to depressive states. One particular study even goes so far as to state "that PCOS is induced by psychological distress and episodes of overeating and/or dieting during puberty and adolescence, when body dissatisfaction and emotional distress are often present." Women with PCOS often have a history of disordered eating, and this study has shown how interconnected stress and eating disorders are and how they can lead to PCOS because of the dysregulation of the cortisol-glucose-insulin relationship. This patient had anorexia during her early years of puberty, which changed her hormonal story for a long time.

This patient that I am speaking to you about is me.

There was a pivotal moment in my life that woke me up to the disordered state that I had been living in; it was when my best friend suddenly died in an accident. That shock, that level of grief, forced me to reassess my life and how I was living it. I knew my body had been speaking to me for a long time. I knew I had suppressed emotions and traumas I needed to deal with that had dictated so many of my decisions. Going into my grief allowed me to make life-changing decisions and see truths I had tucked away in my subconscious for a long time. I left my then husband, I decided to travel the world after graduating naturopathic medical school and knew it was time to heal.

For me, grief and sadness gave me space to finally feel happiness. A happiness that now comes from a knowing that my inner critic isn't my voice, nor does it speak truth. A knowing that the sadness I still often feel doesn't have to overwhelm me but can inform me. This relationship with depression I feel will be a lifelong one. It shows up in different ways and even more intensely now in perimenopause. Knowing that my hormonal changes will impact this feeling and how much control it has over me gives me the capacity to use the tools I know and have, to use this state to heal more layers of my story. Using the HER Method and having my nonnegotiable habits, nutrients, and practices every day have allowed me to continue healing. I may still stumble and have new and interesting symptoms show up now in my 40s, but the more love I pour into my hormones and myself, the more love I can pour into healing myself, my relationships, and my life.

## Hormonal Rage

Anger and extreme irritability are common during the luteal phase and perimenopause, affecting women worldwide. These emotions not only disrupt how women feel but also strain their relationships, creating both internal and external conflict. The root of this anger has multiple layers and can offer valuable insights into habits, thoughts, and unresolved stories that need attention and healing.

Hormonal fluctuations, particularly low levels of progesterone and estrogen, play a significant role in these feelings. However, an inflamed body and brain can also create a hostile physical environment, leading to heightened emotional responses. Anger, while often uncomfortable, can serve as a catalyst for change. It invites you to reflect on where your personal boundaries have been crossed, both in the past and present.

One of the most significant barriers to hormonal healing is being stuck in a pattern of people-pleasing or struggling to say no. Many women spend years prioritizing the needs of others over their own, which can eventually lead to resentment and anger. Over time, the inability to express your needs builds up, becoming stored in the body and organs. This suppressed anger often surfaces more intensely when hormone levels drop and the protective buffer they provide fades away.

Anger can be a powerful motivator for change, but when we stay stuck in it, it contributes to a harmful cycle of inflammation and low immunity by increasing proinflammatory cytokines like interleukin-6 (IL-6). A study exploring the link between anger and IL-6 examined how social support might help reduce the negative effects of this cytokine, which perpetuates the cycle of anger, inflammation, and disease.

What stood out in the study was how it distinguished anger from anxiety. From an evolutionary perspective, anger is an "approach" emotion, pushing us to confront challenges, whereas fear and anxiety are "avoidance" emotions, prompting us to flee or freeze. Anger, compared to anxiety, was found to result in higher cardiac output and lower cortisol reactivity, keeping us more grounded in the present and preparing us for action. In contrast, anxiety pulls us into retreat or immobilization.

The study also highlighted the importance of social support in reducing the connection between anger, inflammation, and disease. This reaffirms something we've always known: Humans need connection. Community isn't just emotional support—it's physical medicine. Without it, we don't just feel isolated; our bodies feel the impact too.

"I don't know what you're doing with her, but I finally have my wife back." I had been working with a woman for a few months, and one day while at a park with my kids, her husband approached me, saying how thankful he was for the work we were doing. For months they had been having arguments routinely, a week before her period. From his perspective, suddenly it was like she had transformed into this fiery, reactive, anger-filled woman that had no resemblance to the wife he had always known. His wife had recently turned 42, and he'd noticed that everything had changed.

After testing her hormones, it became clear that her progesterone was completely depleted, her estrogen was out of balance, and her testosterone was lower than normal. To make matters worse, her body was converting testosterone into 5-alpha dihydrotestosterone (DHT), an enzyme linked to hair loss and low libido. Physically, she felt as though her body was betraying her, and emotionally, she believed that nothing ever went her way. She was stuck in a job she didn't want and felt utterly drained on every level.

Culturally, she had grown up in a household where children had little say in their future. Becoming a doctor or lawyer were the only acceptable career paths, and she had been raised with the belief that her primary duty as a woman was to support her husband, care for her children, and always be there for extended family and friends. She'd never felt she had a choice in her own life, so she sought significance by being the one everyone could rely on, often sacrificing her own health and desires in the process.

But then perimenopause hit, and her body started saying no for her. She could no longer suppress her feelings or needs, but because she was out of practice expressing herself, her emotions often surfaced as aggressive anger. She was exhausted and felt completely "done." Once we worked on improving her physical health through the HER Method and addressing the patterns in her relationships, she was able to calm her nervous system. This allowed her to communicate in a way that was not only assertive and clear but also kind.

Healing our hormones gives us an opportunity to heal so many parts of ourselves; the past, present, and future versions of ourselves get to step into a place of power while dissolving all the entanglements that keep us stuck. Your emotions don't have to control you or your actions but can support your inquiry into your hormonal health to live a more vital and energized life.

## GUIDED MEDITATION: RELEASING RESENTMENT & RECLAIMING YOUR POWER

This meditation will help you access the courage to say no without guilt, release resentment and unexpressed anger, and create space for emotional healing and hormonal balance. Unspoken needs and swallowed emotions—especially anger and frustration—can build up as hormonal rage, anxiety, or exhaustion. This practice allows you to set healthy boundaries and reclaim your energy. Find a quiet space where you feel safe and supported. Sit or lie down, close your eyes, and take a deep breath. Inhale through your nose . . . hold for a moment . . . and exhale slowly through your mouth.

### Step 1: Grounding into Your Strength

Imagine yourself standing in the middle of a vast, open field. The earth beneath you is strong, solid, and unwavering. With every inhale, you draw in strength from the earth. With every exhale, you release any tension, fear, or guilt. A gentle but powerful wind begins to move through the field, brushing against your skin. This wind carries away the heaviness of old obligations and expectations. You whisper to yourself:

"I am safe in my body. My boundaries are sacred."

### Step 2: Meeting the Voice of Your Boundaries

In the distance, you see a version of yourself standing tall and confident. She moves with ease, speaks with clarity, and radiates self-respect. She has no hesitation in saying no when it is necessary. She does not shrink, overexplain, or feel guilty for taking care of herself.

She looks at you with warmth and strength and says:

"You are allowed to say no. You are allowed to protect your energy. No is not rejection—it is self-respect."

You step closer to her and notice she is holding a heavy bag. This bag represents all the times you said yes when you wanted to say no, all the resentment you have carried for taking on too much.

She hands you the bag and asks:

"Are you ready to put this down?"

You pause and feel into your body. Are you ready to let it go?

Inhale deeply . . . and as you exhale, you drop the bag to the ground.

You watch as it dissolves into the earth, leaving you feeling lighter, stronger, and free.

### Step 3: Releasing Hormonal Rage & Resentment

Now bring your attention to your throat and chest. This is where unspoken emotions often get stuck—where the words you never said, the boundaries you never set, and the anger you suppressed live. Imagine a warm, golden light beginning to glow in this area, melting away tension, opening your voice, and clearing blocked emotions. Place your hand over your heart and whisper:

"I release the anger that is not mine to carry."

"My voice matters. My needs matter."

"Saying no is an act of love—for myself and others."

Inhale deeply . . . and exhale with a sigh, releasing any lingering resentment.

### Step 4: Claiming Your Boundaries with Confidence

Picture yourself surrounded by a glowing shield of golden light. This shield represents your boundaries. It is strong but flexible, open but protective. It lets in love, joy, and connection while keeping out energy that drains you.

Now visualize a moment in your life where you need to say no. Maybe it's an overwhelming commitment, a toxic relationship, or a pattern of overgiving. See yourself in that moment, standing tall, confident, and calm. As you speak, your voice is steady and clear:

"No, I cannot do that."

"That does not work for me."

"I love myself too much to say yes to this."

The energy around you shifts. The world does not fall apart. Instead, you feel freer, lighter, and stronger.

Inhale deeply . . . and as you exhale, feel the peace that comes with honoring yourself.

### Step 5: Returning to the Present with Renewed Power

The strong, confident version of yourself looks at you and says:

"You have always had this power inside you. Now it is time to use it."

She places her hand on your shoulder, and as she does, her energy merges into yours.

You are now one with this strong, boundary-honoring version of yourself.

You turn back toward your golden path, walking forward with ease, grace, and certainty.

Inhale deeply . . . and exhale, anchoring this strength into your body.

Slowly wiggle your fingers and toes, bring awareness back to your space, and open your eyes.

## Reflection & Integration

After this meditation, take a few moments to journal your experience. Ask yourself:

- Where in my life do I need stronger boundaries?
- What emotions came up as I imagined saying no?
- What is one small way I can honor myself today?

**Remember:** Saying no does not mean rejecting others—it means **choosing yourself**. The more you honor your own needs, the more **peace, stability, and hormonal balance** you will create in your life.

**You are strong. You are worthy. You are allowed to take up space.**

CHAPTER 6

# Accepting HER, in Every Stage

A woman's life unfolds in three distinct seasons, each with its own rhythm, lessons, and purpose.

The Curiosity Phase spans from birth to puberty, a time when she is wide-eyed and open, soaking in her environment. During these early years, she learns by observing her family and those around her, absorbing the unspoken nuances of what it means to be a woman.

The Vitality Phase takes her from puberty to menopause. This is a period of growth, exploration, and external influence. Here, she wrestles with questions of identity—*Who am I? Who am I meant to be?*—often prioritizing the needs of others over her own. She is shaped by the expectations of peers and society, navigating the balance between giving and self-discovery.

Finally, the Wise Woman Phase begins at menopause and lasts through the rest of her life. This is a time of deep reflection, when she turns inward to rediscover her true self. Freed from external pressures, she lets go of outdated beliefs and embraces the wisdom and authenticity she has carried all along.

The Vitality Phase is when a woman should feel her most energized and excited for life, full of strength and possibility. Yet, for many, the reality is far different. Everyday stress and reproductive challenges, like menstrual issues and fertility struggles, often drain that vitality. This phase, meant to be a time of empowerment, can leave women feeling anything but powerful, challenging the transition into the Wise Woman Phase. That loss of power, I believe, is a result of our loss of connection to our bodies, especially our menstrual cycle.

*Shakti*, a Sanskrit word meaning "power," refers to the unique, transformative energy women hold during their menstrual cycle. In ancient cultures, this time of bleeding was seen as a sacred opportunity for women to release the emotional and physical burdens of the previous month, allowing them to reconnect with themselves and nature.

For example, the goddess Kamakhya Devi is honored in a temple in India, celebrating this powerful gift women possess. Historically, women were given time for solitude during their cycle to rest, cleanse, and heal. However, this view of menstruation as sacred has shifted over time. Instead of being seen as a time of restoration, menstruation has come to be viewed as inconvenient and even impure in many societies. In modern Western culture, women are often pressured to suppress their connection with their bodies during this time, driven by the demands of competition, success, and achievement. The powerful, healing aspects of menstruation have been overshadowed by narratives of pain and inconvenience.

The key concept here is the reclaiming of menstruation as a sacred, empowering experience rather than a societal burden. By shifting the perception toward menstruation, women can reconnect with their own inner power, honor the cyclical nature of their bodies, and embrace this time for rest, rejuvenation, and healing, once again connecting to their vitality.

## The Power of Perception

How women have been perceived in society is dependent on a few factors. Religion, culture, economic and social status, geography, and, I also believe, the stories and beliefs a woman heard growing up about herself and how they turned into her inner voice. The reverence toward women, one could say, changed drastically with the rise of a world where men began to desire power more than connection. In some sources it is said that this change started around 3,000 to 3,500 years ago, where the cultural perception of a woman's role changed. Before this time, in most cultures, a woman was seen as a man's equal and even revered for the relationship she had with nature. She was seen to be able to wield the powers of nature through her connection to the earth and moon cycles. She was given the gift to create life and, according to Chinese medicine, carries the essence or chi (energy) of Mother Earth. It was said that during menstruation, a woman was ready to be a spirit medium, a vessel to source itself. When this shifted into believing that bleeding was due to some sort of punishment or curse, or that it was a form of pollution, or completely unsacred and dirty, so did the behavior toward women, creating the imprints of trauma and perceptions of who we are supposed to be, an identity we carry with us even today.

How we have been perceived and how women have been treated in the medical system when it comes to their reproductive health clearly needs to change to heal these imprints. To be constantly told your symptoms are all in your head, or to feel like you don't want to be a bother so you keep your discomforts to yourself, or when you feel like all you can do is hide from the world because of the overwhelm, these scenarios, whether external or internal, validate those old beliefs and keep you in a state of forgetting and rejection of your power and your purpose: to be the awesome goddess that you truly are. The healing starts with you. By changing your own relationship with your body, emotions, and hormones. When we begin to feel the wisdom we carry in our womb and the gift we are given every month, that is when we will start to truly rewrite our story. Menopause will no longer be feared, your period will no longer be a threat to your lifestyle or relationships, and we will no longer need approval from the outside world to be the vivacious viragos we truly are (a virago is a woman that dares to challenge societal norms with some sass and some style)! Change your perception and free yourself from the chains of society and your mind. Not only will this start the healing journey toward healing your relationship with yourself, but also with others.

There is a Taoist teaching on perception about the lord of Wei and a beautiful woman he favored and spent time with. The lord had strict rules about his carriage and had declared that anyone who used it without his permission would be punished by getting their foot chopped off (yikes!). One day Mi Tzu-hsia, the beautiful woman, heard about her mother falling ill and took the carriage without his permission to go see her. In his eyes, she did an act of devotion and took such a risk for her mother and therefore should be praised for it. On another day they were both on a walk, and Mi Tzu-hsia had pulled a peach off a tree, bit into its juiciness, and gave the rest to the lord. He praised her once again, thinking she had sacrificed her pleasure so he could experience it himself. Years went by and Mi Tzu-hsia started to get older and was losing her youthful vitality and beauty and no longer was in his favor. There was an incident where she had done something to offend him, and in his new perception of her, he stated, "I remember how she once took my carriage without my permission. And another time she gave me a peach that she had already bitten into!" and here, his love for her began to fade. One simple change in his perception of her changed everything.

After reading this story, take a moment to reflect on your own monthly cycle. Whether you still menstruate or not, you're still connected to the cycles of the moon and the women around you who do, so this applies to everyone. Think about your close relationships: Are there times in the month when you feel connected and positive toward others, where even their annoying habits don't bother you, and you let things slide easily? And then, are there moments when those same habits suddenly irritate you, triggering a wave of frustration or even anger you didn't know you had? In those moments, your perception shifts, and you might start creating a story about who that person is, reshaping your relationship—not toward love and growth, but toward resentment and distance.

Just as the lord in the Tao story experienced a shift in perception, our hormonal and emotional changes can strongly influence how we see our relationships. Add modern stressors and fluctuating hormones, and it's easy to get stuck in a distorted view of those connections.

Twelve years ago, a couple came to our clinic, seeking hormonal help. I worked with the wife while my husband treated her husband. After running tests and understanding why she felt so hopeless, lost, and disconnected from her body and life, we developed a plan. We helped her manage stress, reduce inflammation through better food choices, and explore the emotions she had toward her husband.

She discovered patterns from her upbringing that were showing up in her marriage. In her effort to avoid becoming like her mother, she had developed a hard exterior, leaning heavily into her masculine energy. She prided herself on being emotionally and financially self-reliant, never needing to rely on her husband. But this mindset created a type A personality—constantly in control, unable to trust others, and always busy because "no one could do things as well as she could." This stress-driven lifestyle disrupted her hormones, leaving her nurturing side on the sidelines.

By her 40s, during perimenopause, this approach no longer served her. She was exhausted, had no sex drive, felt bloated daily, lost chunks of hair, and suffered from migraines before her period. Over several months, we worked together to heal the inner child who had made the decision to shut down parts of herself to feel safe. We focused on reconnecting her with those missing pieces while improving her physical symptoms using bioidentical hormones. This gave her the energy and space to address the unresolved traumas she had been avoiding for so long.

As we did this work, her husband worked on himself too. Eventually, we stopped seeing them, but months later, a friend of theirs came in for treatment and told us, "I don't think you realize, but you helped save a marriage." Hearing those words was a powerful reminder of how important this work is. It showed me how quickly we can lose so much in our lives because of our emotional state in a single moment. But just as one moment can lead to life-altering decisions, one moment can also lead to life-healing choices.

The Curiosity Phase and Vitality Phase play a significant role in shaping how smooth or challenging your transition into perimenopause and menopause will be. The experiences and stories from these phases influence your beliefs, habits, hormones, and emotions as you undergo this transformation—affecting not just your body and mind but also your relationships. Remember, the healing work you do isn't just for you; it benefits your entire family.

## The Aging Brain

"Doc, I'm losing it!" a woman told me one day, frustrated by how often she walked into a room and forgot why she was there. She couldn't focus, kept forgetting names, and felt like her brain was declining too quickly. We've all felt scattered under stress, struggling to focus or remember things. For many women in perimenopause or menopause, issues with short-term memory are a common and concerning complaint.

As estrogen levels drop, the brain's ability to create neural connections in the memory and learning centers weakens, making it harder to do simple tasks like remembering where you left your keys. This symptom is particularly scary for women, because many of us have witnessed loved ones battle Alzheimer's or dementia, and we know the devastating impact it can have on families.

Out of all the losses in my life, losing my nani, my maternal grandmother, was the hardest. She had endured significant trauma, and when my nana, her husband, passed away, it seemed like her brain couldn't handle it anymore. She quickly slipped into dementia. Watching someone you love lose themselves and their memories is indescribably painful, and I know many of you reading this can relate. It's a long, emotional journey filled with moments of both sorrow and joy.

Knowing this was part of my family's story, I became deeply curious about dementia—what causes it and how it connects to hormonal health. I discovered the term *dementogens* (sounds like something out of Harry Potter, right?), which refers to toxins that contribute to dementia. These same toxins—like heavy metals (lead, aluminum, mercury), harmful chemicals in cosmetics and cleaners, and biotoxins in food—can also disrupt hormonal balance. This confirmed for me that healing our hormones can protect both body and brain as we age.

As we grow older, our natural decline in hormones leaves us more vulnerable to stress—whether emotional, chemical, or physical. By perimenopause and menopause, our brain's protective layer is compromised, so caring for brain health becomes essential. Understanding how your life story and hormonal history from your previous phases affect your brain can help you see how these changes impact your emotions and relationships.

This awareness provides an opportunity to use tools from the HER Method to support your brain and body as you enter this new chapter of life—the Wise Woman Phase. So, let me reassure you: You're not losing your marbles. Your brain is simply responding to its environment, giving you a chance to heal, grow, and unlock the wisdom within.

## The Power of Letting Go

Aging is a difficult topic for many of us, especially if we've witnessed loved ones struggle physically, emotionally, or mentally as they've grown older. It's even harder in a world that constantly pushes the message to fight aging at all costs. But what if we reframed aging as a gift?

I know it's not easy to feel that way when your body seems to be betraying you or when your mind feels less sharp than it once was. However, with the understanding you now have about how your hormones and life story influence your body, I hope you can see the power you hold. You have the ability to support your body and brain in aging gracefully, embracing each phase with strength and wisdom.

In recent years, there has been increased awareness about menopause, aging, and the challenges women face during this phase of life. However, what's often overlooked is the transition phase before menopause: perimenopause. Much like puberty, perimenopause can leave women feeling lost—disconnected from their bodies, overwhelmed by shifting emotions, and unsure about relationships they once felt secure in.

The key difference between puberty and perimenopause is that puberty feels like a beginning—a step toward adulthood, where the world is full of opportunities to explore, create, and dream. Perimenopause, on the other hand, can feel like a loss—losing a sense of self, losing the hormonal rhythm that once anchored your identity, and losing the ability to dream big. For many, it's a time filled with symptoms like joint pain, hot flashes, insomnia, and more, leading to the perception that life is now on a downward slope.

But what if we could shift that perception? What if, like our teenage years, perimenopause could be seen as a time of transformation, an opportunity to rediscover and recreate ourselves? Free from the societal expectations of who we're supposed to be, we gain the freedom to choose who we want to become.

Perimenopause is much like the transition phase in labor—when your entire body shakes, and you feel completely out of control. But then, in the moment you finally surrender, a beautiful baby is born. In that intense, uncertain moment, a new version of yourself is being birthed, asking you to let go of who you thought you needed to be, who society and family told you to be, and to embrace this new chapter of life.

Similarly, during perimenopause, as your hormones shift, your future wise-woman self—the one who emerges after menopause—is calling on you to release old identities. This might mean letting go of the body you once knew, the life you were comfortable with, or the thought patterns you've clung to for so long. However, this transition can feel especially difficult if there are unresolved emotions or unfinished healing that need your attention.

Perimenopause brings a mix of emotions: grief for what is passing, joy for what is to come, rage at the upheaval, and excitement for the possibilities ahead. You may notice changes not only in your inner world but also in your outer life—children growing and leaving home, a shift in how you approach your work, or new priorities around who and what you spend your time on. By supporting your hormones during this time, you can help your body and brain navigate this transition more smoothly, allowing you to step into this new phase with greater ease and grace.

## The Power of Acceptance

Aging is not just a biological process; it's also a cultural one. The society and culture we grow up in play a significant role in shaping our feelings about aging, often creating anxiety around it. Many women experience shame as their bodies go through changes that feel unfamiliar or difficult to understand. Even women in their 20s are already worried about how they'll look in the future, spending time and money on Botox and fillers—not to embrace beauty but out of fear of societal rejection. They're led to believe that aging means losing value, worth, and the ability to live a full life filled with adventure, curiosity, and love, all because of the physical changes in their bodies. But what if we could see aging differently—as the body maturing and ripening to match the wisdom of the soul?

My nani used to say, "Look at my hands. They've changed so much. They used to be so young, and now they look so old," with a smile and a little giggle. I wish I had asked her more questions about her childhood and what she had learned through the years. I wish I had given her the space to tell her stories and share how she saw herself as her body and mind changed. Even after decades of serving her family, her wrinkles, graying hair, achy knees, and occasional sharp words for my nana when he interrupted her favorite soap opera, her eyes still sparkled with youthful curiosity and mischief. She taught me what it looks like to embrace aging—finding joy in simple, everyday moments and appreciating the present. Even as dementia began to take her further from us, every time I looked into her eyes, I could still see her: the wise woman, the sage who shared her wisdom through her presence. She showed me that old age doesn't have to be resisted but accepted as a natural and beautiful part of life.

It's our resistance to aging that creates suffering and pain. In acceptance, we gain access to the wisdom we've cultivated through our hormonal and emotional journeys. The way we view ourselves and our experiences shapes how we navigate perimenopause and menopause. Remember, the symptoms you feel are your body's language, and the emotions you experience are your soul's voice. Together, they guide you to understand what you truly need.

The discomfort and challenges in your body and relationships often intensify because it's time to release old wounds and unfinished stories from the past. As these resurface, your body speaks—through physical aches, emotional pain, or even new awareness of long-standing issues. A study from Project Viva at Harvard Medical School, which followed 682 women over 20 years, found that those who experienced childhood abuse—whether physical, emotional, sexual, or financial—faced more severe menopausal symptoms. This shows us how unresolved trauma, carried into new stages of life, requires focused support for the nervous system and stress hormones to break free from the cycle of hypervigilance and chronic stress.

The stress patterns imprinted in the brain, the loss of hormonal protection in areas like memory and emotion, and the shift in how you process the world can trigger physical responses—pelvic pain, inflamed joints, or stubborn belly weight—that won't fully resolve until you release the stored emotions and heal the hormonal and neural imbalances behind them. In the coming chapters, you'll learn tools and techniques to help your body and brain release these patterns, rewire your systems, and move forward into healing.

## From Wild Woman to Wise Woman

In the women I've supported through menopause, I've observed something beautiful: Those who embrace self-awareness and self-acceptance develop a humility that allows them to befriend aging. They come to recognize that this stage of life is their time to focus on themselves. While they may confront fears about mortality—especially as loved ones face illness or aging—and navigate the shifting dynamics of their relationships with children or aging parents, they also realize the freedom that comes from aligning with their soul's calling. By connecting more deeply with themselves and the divine, they begin to release the daily stressors that once weighed them down.

I call this the "no f***s given" stage. The chaos and complexity of the reproductive years transform into a state where women care less about what others think and more about how they feel and think about themselves. This shift has a profound impact on their health and relationships. Imagine how freeing that must feel!

What I would love to see is more open conversations about aging between younger women and those moving through later phases of life. Imagine being 25 and hearing from a confident, unapologetic 55-year-old woman who loves who she is and celebrates her aging body. Imagine receiving wisdom about how to prepare for the hormonal and life transitions ahead—how to care for yourself in body, mind, and spirit. This kind of mentorship could create a world filled with women who confidently speak their truth, heal generational wounds, and live vibrant, peaceful lives, even amid chaos.

The principles of healing are universal, whether you're in your reproductive years, navigating perimenopause, or stepping into menopause. That said, how we eat, move, think, and approach daily habits must evolve as our hormones change. This journey will look different for every woman, but the foundation remains the same: Know yourself and identify the factors that disrupt your inner harmony. Certain systems in your body will require more care during this time, and prioritizing the health of your nervous system that you will learn in the HER Method is key to rewriting the patterns of trauma and stress imprinted in your hormonal story.

## Loneliness and the Gifts of Aging

Many menopausal women report a sense of doom—a wave of panic that sometimes precedes physical symptoms like hot flashes. This unsettling feeling can serve as a window of opportunity to reflect on their relationship with their body and the unresolved stress still gripping their nervous system. The beauty of this phase is that, for many women, there is finally time. With careers more established and children growing more independent, they may shift from micromanaging others' lives to focusing on their own personal growth—though this shift often comes with a layer of grief as they let go of familiar roles.

One of the most challenging adjustments women face during menopause, alongside physical changes, is the shift in their relationships, particularly with their partners. After years of prioritizing family and careers, many couples find themselves living parallel lives, simply managing the day-to-day. But when the busyness subsides, women often realize they need to relearn how to connect with their partners on a deeper level. Without supporting the nervous system, this process can feel overwhelming. Hormonal changes can create inner chaos, making it harder to meet their partners emotionally, which can lead to feelings of loneliness and disconnection.

Loneliness is a recurring theme I see in so many women's lives, and it deeply impacts both emotional and physical health. A 2016 study found that individuals who reported loneliness had more amyloid plaques—proteins associated with Alzheimer's and dementia—in their brains compared to those who didn't feel lonely. Reflecting on my nani's journey with dementia, I often wonder how the loss of her husband, the love of her life, contributed to her cognitive decline. Feeling alone in her pain and trauma may have significantly affected her brain health.

Loneliness also raises stress-hormone levels, triggering inflammation and increasing the risk of disease. For menopausal women, who are already at higher risk of cardiovascular issues due to declining estrogen, loneliness compounds the danger by raising blood pressure and weakening the immune system. It even alters the brain's neurochemistry, reducing dopamine-receptor activity and making it harder to feel joy—something already strained during this stage due to lower hormone levels.

Women today feel even more isolated because of society's obsession with antiaging and its lack of open conversation about the real changes happening in their bodies and minds. This silence leaves many women feeling disconnected from themselves and the people they love.

Physical changes like vaginal dryness, lower libido, and hot flashes can also make emotional and physical intimacy with partners difficult. Many menopausal women feel resentful after spending so many years caregiving for their families and partners. When these women start to express their needs and opinions, their partners may struggle to adjust, as they haven't been preparing for this transition in the same way the women in their lives have. Involving your partner in the journey can foster understanding and strengthen your relationship.

Let's be real—it would be great if our loved ones could read our minds! But in my experience, couples who support each other's healing build healthier, more connected relationships. Women, however, are often unaccustomed to voicing their needs. For generations, we've been taught to prioritize others, making it difficult to ask for or receive love and care.

Entering the Wise Woman Phase requires learning to set boundaries and embrace the art of receiving. While this may feel unfamiliar, asking for help—whether from the people in your life or from the divine—is a vital part of healing. By including yourself in your prayers and focusing on your own well-being, you begin to reconnect with your innate value and worth. You tap into the wisdom passed down through generations of women before you, grounding yourself in your identity and strength.

As you embrace this power, you become the wise woman you've always known you could be, unapologetically using your gifts to guide and inspire the next generation. This, my sister, is how we change the world—one prayer, one empowered woman at a time.

No matter which phase of life you're in, healing is a choice you can make. The next few chapters will guide you through your **hormonal** journey, helping you find peace within your body and **emotions** while strengthening your **relationships.**

PART II

# The HER Method

## A Proven Method to Heal Hormonal Chaos and Emotional Overload

CHAPTER 7

# Hierarchy of Hormonal Healing

*The greatest form of self-care and self-love is to know thyself.* If we gave the same devotion we have for others to ourselves, our health would never sit in limbo or in the unknown. We would have full awareness of how we feel. We would be aware of where the feelings come from and what they are trying to tell us. These layers of healing we move through ask women to step into the wilderness of their physical and emotional body and, most importantly, their story. It asks us to commit to fully seeing ourselves as the powerhouse and wisdom holders we are. Here we dive into the why behind the state of stress that impacts our hormones and how this state has taken away the very thing women need to heal, self-trust. We start to unlock the mystery behind the reactions, the sometimes edginess toward our partner, the sadness in the alone moments, and the inner rage that has had no place to go. To look through an emotional lens on healing so you can re-establish trust in yourself, in your body, and in your emotions. There are three key areas that need your attention: self-respect, self-awareness, and self-initiation. This is what I refer to as the Triangle of Hormonal Empowerment, a concept that can help you understand why healing your hormones, emotions, and relations can be challenging and how easily we can unstick ourselves from the chaos and challenge when we understand the power of the triangle.

One of the action steps one must take to initiate this triangle of empowerment is understanding your relationship with boundaries. Are there times in your life when you feel like you have trouble saying no or trouble using your voice to relay what is important to you? When boundaries are fluid out of fear—fear of not belonging, fear of losing love, or fear of being called out and being different—it slowly removes the trust we have for ourselves and challenges this concept of *self-respect*. Learning how to skillfully say no creates the opportunity to say yes to something or someone else.

Saying no to a new project opportunity that on the surface sounds amazing but is something you lack passion for and will take up a lot of your time, will allow you to say yes to perhaps time with your family or time to pursue a project you are passionate about. Learning to say yes to others even when we know it will deplete us is often a learned behavior from the women around us, or out of necessity to feel accepted and loved.

As we've learned, living without boundaries can unknowingly foster resentment—toward others and even yourself. This resentment, in turn, can disrupt both your hormonal and relational health. Unfortunately, our society doesn't model or teach healthy boundaries well. Instead, those who say yes are often praised, and women, in particular, are expected to comply. When the time comes to prioritize healthy boundaries, it requires significant unlearning and deconditioning. Establishing boundaries is a vital step in building a strong relationship with self-worth and self-respect, both of which are essential for deep healing and owning your story.

## Triangle of Hormonal Empowerment

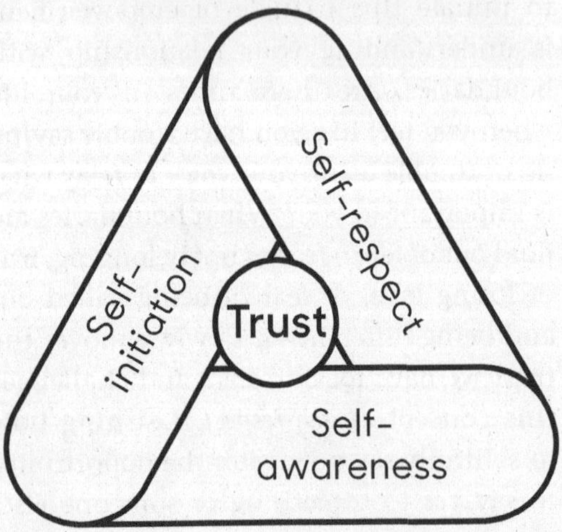


**Self-respect** can be defined in many ways; I see it as faith in oneself. The worth one puts on their values and commitments, and I see it as the foundation of self-love and self-acceptance. When you respect yourself, you can trust yourself. When you trust yourself, you know the decisions you will make, the actions you will take will lead to your growth and healing. When you trust yourself, you know then that the emotions you are feeling are telling you a story and are a gateway to your soul's whispers that will always lead you to your truth and to what you need. Trust is the source of energy that oxytocin relies on to help you feel connected, feel like you belong, and feel loved.

*How would you describe trust or what it feels like to know that trust exists?*

Trust can be felt as an embodied feeling in all your cells. It is a feeling in your gut and in your heart that all will be well. There is a warmth and comfort in this feeling that is unshakable no matter what the external circumstance may be. It is a feeling that allows you to pause, reflect, and then act. It is a feeling you can access easily when the chaos of stress in your body is removed. Self-respect is one leg of the triangle, serving as the anchor that helps you return to trust.

**Self-awareness** forms another leg, guiding you back to that trust. This awareness—of your reactions, stressors, triggers, and the ways your true self may hide—puts the power of choice back in your hands. For example, when you recognize that your progesterone levels drop a week before your cycle, leading to heightened anxiety, you can understand that your reaction to a partner's comment may be amplified by hormonal shifts, not rooted in reality. In that moment, you have the choice to respond thoughtfully rather than react impulsively. This builds trust in your awareness and fosters calm in your relationships.

The concept of self-awareness will be explored further so you can fully embrace and embody its transformative power.

Lastly, **self-initiation**, the will that keeps you in your trust. Initiating oneself into healing is the very thing that will keep you curious, growing, and even humble through the process of self-discovery. When you take the steps toward inquiry about why you feel as you do and how it has impacted your life, you create a silent contract with your soul. Or perhaps you unveil one that had already existed to continuously stay on this path even when you feel stuck.

The will to keep going is essential, especially when life throws you a curveball just as you've found your rhythm—your ideal diet, an exercise routine your body loves, and the tools that make you feel vital and like yourself again. Suddenly, you're pulled back into a memory, a trigger, or a deep state of stress, grief, anger, or sadness. It's this self-initiation and inner will that remind you: This is temporary, and it, too, shall pass.

When you are self-initiated, your drive for healing comes from an intrinsic desire and motivation that keeps you in the long game. We are conditioned to look outside of ourselves, to other supposed experts on our own bodies. Asking for help, learning from others, and finding wisdom in our elders is necessary for us to uncover our own ability to heal; it is when we expect the other to heal us that we subconsciously tell ourselves we can't trust our own intuition and judgment. Sometimes we need a nudge in the right direction, but a true healer helps you remember along the way that it was your ability to initiate yourself onto this path that will bring you the healing you need. Self-initiation helps you initiate self-discipline to stay on course toward that vital self you imagined you could be, full of life, energy, and love toward yourself and everyone around you. Where there is discipline, there is trust; where there is trust, there is access to joy.

## The HER Method Hierarchy of Hormonal Healing

"I finally feel like myself. I finally feel in control of my health and my life." These are the words I love hearing when women tap into their innate healing and discover that there are solutions to their discomforts. When they first come to see me, it's often because of physical symptoms. But over time, they realize that while these symptoms show up in the body, true healing also requires addressing the relational, mental, and emotional aspects of their lives. Only then can their whole self truly heal. Those that are able and willing to become more self-aware in the end realize all that work eventually leads them back to their inner healer that was there all along; it was the noise of life, old beliefs, and the various stressors that were getting in the way of them hearing what she had to say.

Healing your hormones involves many layers. It can feel overwhelming to process all the information and implement the necessary changes, but true healing happens when you address the root cause rather than just placing a Band-Aid on the symptoms.

Below is the system of hierarchy that I like to work from to help women ease into the journey. If I can help a woman feel even a little bit better physically, it creates more room to look deeper into the emotional and all the other layers in her life. Let's take a deeper dive into what to look for in each layer and how you can use this information to start making changes now! This chapter will lay out the foundation for healing before we get into the protocols in the coming chapters on what day-to-day healing can look like. These strategies are meant to empower you with the questions and insights you can take to your doctor and the tests you need to ask your doctor about to better implement these solutions, while also giving you tools you can incorporate right away.

## The Physical Level

As we've learned in previous chapters, hormones respond to their environment—both the internal environment within the body and the external environment surrounding the cells. These environments are shaped by various stressors, including physical, chemical, and emotional ones. When I begin treating women, my first step is to identify the stressors in their environment that might be blocking their healing.

### Hierarchy of Hormonal Healing

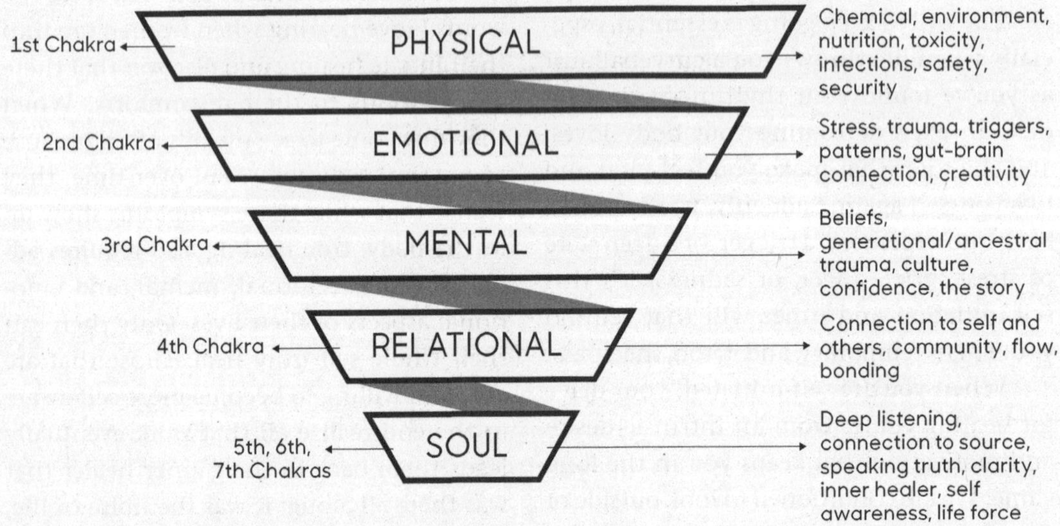

This includes examining factors like heavy metals, mold, dormant or active infections, parasites, genetic predispositions, and nutritional deficiencies, as well as anything that threatens a woman's physical safety or security.

Healing can feel nearly impossible when you're exhausted, in pain, unable to focus, or disconnected from your body. To heal emotionally, we must first address the physical, creating the energy and capacity needed for deeper work. Over the years, I've seen that when a woman feels physically better, there's nothing she can't do. Emotional healing feels less overwhelming, because healing the body naturally begins to heal the mind.

These stressors trigger a cascade of reactions in her body that includes changes in her hormonal and reproductive health. In the previous chapters, we spent time understanding how your body holds on to your story in different organs and systems. When trying to heal this story from a physical perspective, I make sure to check all the boxes for testing all that influences the physical but also paying equal attention to the emotions and energetics of the physical body and how it is all connected.

As a yoga teacher and someone who has spent years studying the chakras and their influence on how we navigate life, I find it essential to bridge the gap between the physical and energetic worlds. The connection between these helps women understand the profound power of their physical form and allows them to move toward deeper emotional healing. Recognizing this interplay also provides access to a wider range of healing tools. It shifts the focus from quick fixes—like replacing a medication with a supplement—to adopting a variety of practices and habits that work together to reignite your body's natural healing potential.

The first stage of healing in the hierarchy corresponds to the root chakra (one of the pockets of energy in the body), which is linked to our physical needs and connection to the material world. It represents safety, stability, and grounding—the very things women often feel they've lost when life feels overwhelming. Physically, the root chakra is associated with the uterus, rectum, vagina, and pelvic area, particularly in relation to reproductive health. By understanding this chakra and its connection to your physical health, you will be able to incorporate the tools you will learn in the coming chapters with more intention and a knowing of how it is healing your hormones.

In a 2017 cadaver study, scientists explored the connection between this chakra and its corresponding physical nerve plexus. They examined six cadavers, marking the location of the root chakra, and found it aligned precisely with the inferior hypogastric nerve plexus—a network of nerves that serves specific organs. Interestingly, the triangular shape of this plexus mirrored the symbol of the root chakra (how did they know this thousands of years ago?). The four petals of the chakra symbol may also correspond to its subplexuses: the rectal plexus, spermatic/uterine plexus, vesical plexus, and prostatic/vaginal plexus.

Why is this important? While more research is needed to fully confirm these connections, this study underscores the deep interconnection between your physical body, your personal story, and your emotions. By healing the physical body, you can begin to heal the emotional body, a process you'll explore further in the coming chapters.

When exploring your physical reproductive health, an essential question to ask is: What is jeopardizing or making your sense of safety vulnerable from a physical perspective? What in your environment might be causing harm, and what are you surrounding yourself with that helps you feel grounded and cared for? This can range from the food choices you make to how you move and sleep. It also involves reflecting on the habits from your past—those passed down through generations—and identifying which ones may be blocking your ability to feel good in your body.

To uncover these patterns and create change, there are three key steps: test, track, and transform.

Combining objective **testing** with subjective reflection allows you to uncover what your body has been trying to communicate through its symptoms. On the next pages are some tests that can help reveal your hormonal story and blueprint. While these tests primarily focus on physical symptoms, I've found over the years that they also provide valuable insights into emotional health. They highlight the root causes of the miscommunication and imbalance within your body and hormones, which directly affect your emotional state. For example, feelings of sadness, irritability, or anger before your period may stem from low hormone levels, which, in turn, could be caused by heavy metals blocking your hormones from properly binding to your cells. Without that proper connection, your body can't access the calm and joy that balanced hormones typically provide.

## The 3Ts of Physical Healing

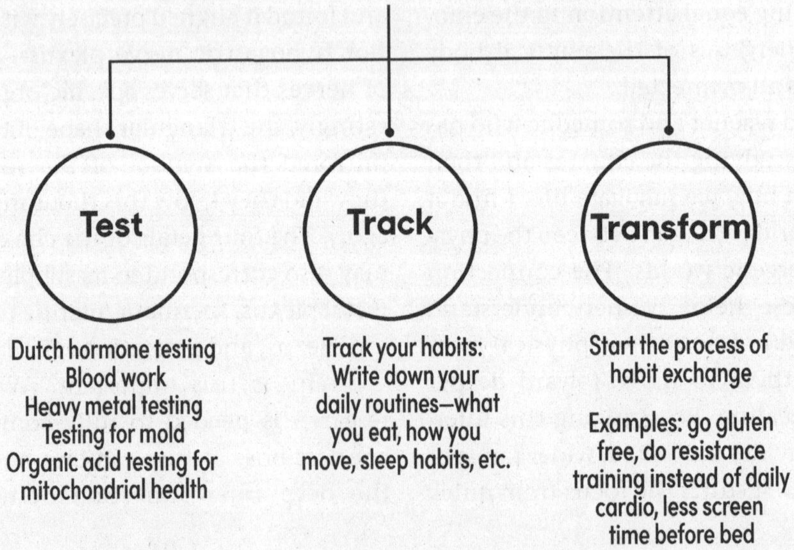

| TEST | WHAT IT IS | WHAT YOU'RE CHECKING | WHY IT'S IMPORTANT |
|---|---|---|---|
| **DUTCH TEST/ HORMONE ZOOMER** | Dry urine test for comprehensive hormone testing | Estrogen, progesterone, testosterone, DHEA, cortisol, melatonin, adrenal health, diurnal rhythm, oxidative stress, nutrient deficiencies, dopamine, liver methylation/detox process, hormone metabolites | Tells you more details around how your body is utilizing your hormones. Breaks down the hormones into their metabolites, giving you more insight into a more focused treatment plan. Diurnal variation and role of adrenals in sleep. |
| **BLOOD WORK** | Testing for inflammation, cardiovascular health, hormones, immune system. Gives you a snapshot into your body. | CBC, ferritin, vitamin D, homocysteine, C-reactive protein, TSH, free T3, free T4, thyroid peroxidase antibody, thyroglobulin, thyroglobulin antibody, uric acid, fasting insulin, hemoglobin A1C, liver enzymes (AST, ALT, GGT), lipid profile, kidney markers (BUN, creatinine), sex hormone-binding globulin, Epstein-Barr virus | Important to have a foundational base of your overall health. When women lose hormones, they are at higher risk for inflammation and a cardiovascular event. This can also give clues as to lingering infections and immune health. |
| **PROVOKED HEAVY METAL URINE TEST (PRE AND POST USING CHELATING AGENTS LIKE DMSA AND INTRAVENOUS EDTA)** | Tests for the most common heavy metals in your environment. | Heavy metals such as mercury, lead, aluminum, arsenic, thallium, etc., and minerals | There are heavy metals in your environment that can get stuck in your tissues, compromising your hormones' ability to do their job. Essentially blocking the hormones and nutrients like minerals uptaken into the cell. This can have a long-term impact on your physical and emotional health. |

| | | | |
|---|---|---|---|
| **ORGANIC ACID TESTING** | Measures organic compounds in your urine that are present because of various biochemical pathways that coordinate your health. | Fungal and bacterial compounds, amino acids, nutrients like vitamin C, B vitamins, glutathione, etc., mitochondrial health (specifically the Krebs cycle, where energy is created), oxalates, neurotransmitter health like serotonin and dopamine pathways | This test gives you deeper insight into your cells. It allows you to understand your mitochondrial health. There are approximately 100,000 mitochondria per mature oocyte. By puberty most young women have 400,000 oocytes. That is a heck of a lot of mitochondria needing to stay healthy to support your reproductive health! |
| **FOOD SENSITIVITY** | Immunoglobulin G (IgG) and immunoglobulin A (IgA) antibody testing against foods | Various foods that you may be sensitive to and have a delayed immune reaction against | The health of your gut determines the health of your hormones and your emotions. Remember, serotonin is made in the gut, if there is inflammation in the gut, your brain and nervous system will not receive the right amount of serotonin to help you feel good. An inflamed gut also prevents detoxification of toxic estrogens in your environment. |
| **IMAGING** | Images of reproductive organs | Ultrasound, transvaginal ultrasound, laparoscopy, etc. | This will depend on what symptoms you are presenting with. Often used for differential diagnosis of, for example, fibroids, cysts, polyps, etc. |
| **OTHERS: MICRONUTRIENT PANELS, DNA TESTING, GUT MICROBIOME TESTING (Gut Zoomer from companies like Vibrant Health)** | Various tests that can be used to further the investigation into your body | These can look at deficiencies in vitamins, minerals, and oils, DNA vulnerabilities, and overall gut health. | These tests are great for maintenance and longevity goals once you have your hormones in check and have uncovered the stressors in the metabolic health bucket that are causing chaos in your hormonal and emotional health. |

**Tracking** your history and your present-day habits can give you more clues to what has been shaping your physical health. This is a great tool to utilize when you start a program so you can see where you are today and how things have changed as you embark on the journey to do the work. Take a moment to write out your health history timeline. This timeline will consist of any significant memory from as far back as you can go. Below is a list of prompts and questions that can help spark some memory for your timeline.

1. What were some health habits that were modeled for you by your family and friends?
2. What have been habits that you created for your health, and what habits did you have that depleted your health?
3. What are some core memories related to stress, joy, loss, health challenges, and victories?
4. What has been your relationship with food in different stages of your life?
5. How have you perceived your body in the past?
6. Did you have any illnesses, surgeries, accidents?
7. How were your emotions received by your caretaker throughout your childhood, and do you have any charge around those memories?
8. What has your reproductive health been like since you started your period?
9. How has your emotional health changed over your reproductive years up until now?
10. What was the messaging you received about health and your body, and what beliefs do you feel you have formed because of it?
11. What are some toxins in your environment that you may have been exposed to growing up?
12. Did you live in an older home that could have had mold? Or work in a building that could have had water damage?
13. Have you noticed any patterns in your health—physical, emotional, or mental?
14. How may these patterns have impacted your relationships?
15. What were the basic pillars of hormonal health like in your past? How did you eat, sleep, or move your body?

After taking some time to reflect on these questions, I encourage you to step back and view your life from an eagle's-eye perspective. This broader view allows you to see all the angles and contributing factors that have shaped the person you are today. Consider how your conditions, experiences, and habits create your present reality.

Is it one of pain and sorrow, joy, acceptance of emotional polarities, contentment and peace, or discomfort and scarcity?

We've learned that the symptoms you experience in your physical body are signals of stress. By tracking your daily habits, choices, and thoughts, you gain insight into where small changes can be made. Over time, these small, consistent adjustments matter far more than occasional efforts. They retrain your body, guiding it toward better health and helping you live free of symptoms.

The Daily Hormone Tracking sheet can be your guide in your present around your habits and your health. Here you can track the basic hormonal health pillars and how they change over the course of your healing.

This habit tracking sheet is designed to do more than simply record your daily actions; it's here to help you see the patterns that shape your hormonal and overall health. By using it regularly, you'll begin to notice which habits support your energy, mood, and cycle, and which ones might be working against your body's natural rhythm.

Each day, take a few moments to check off supportive habits you've completed and note any habits or choices that may be adding stress or creating imbalance. Over time, you'll begin to see clear connections between your routines, your hormones, and how you feel.

The final *T* in your healing journey is **transformation**. After testing and tracking, you've gained insight into your body's unique hormonal patterns and how your symptoms reflect deeper imbalances. Now it's time to take that awareness and turn it into aligned action. Transformation is where knowledge becomes change—where small, intentional shifts in your daily habits begin to create real momentum in your healing. In the chapters ahead, you'll learn how to support your body through nourishing foods, hormone-friendly routines, emotional regulation tools, and deeper connection to your internal rhythms.

## The Emotional Level

The emotional level of healing may require a great deal from you, but I promise, once you embark on this journey, you'll begin to master your life. At this layer, we uncover the hidden stories held within your body and explore how they manifest in your daily life through the lens of your emotions. We'll identify the dominant emotions that shape your mood throughout the month and influence your personality, ultimately affecting how you show up in your closest relationships and how they impact your physical health.

This level is connected to the second chakra, which governs your creativity, sexuality, and emotions. It is associated with the sacral plexus, which controls the function of your bowels, sexual organs, adrenals, and more. When this energy center is balanced, you feel deeply connected to yourself and allow yourself to experience pleasure in your daily life. However, when it's out of balance, many women face reproductive and menstrual challenges caused by stagnant energy—anything from painful intercourse to ovarian cysts.

# Daily Hormone Tracking

SLEEP QUALITY

MOODSCAPE

BOWEL MOVEMENT

MOVEMENT

ENERGY LEVELS

INTENTION FOR THE DAY AND WHAT IS WORKING WELL FOR YOU

Healing this level means repairing one of the most important relationships you will ever have: the one with yourself. You spend every moment with yourself, so nurturing this bond is essential. As you cultivate self-love, you gain the capacity to share that love with others. Many of the stressors and traumas we've discussed in this book reside in this layer. Healing here offers the chance to free yourself from the web of emotional discomfort. As you release these stuck emotions, you'll notice a ripple effect, promoting physical healing as well. Progressing through the hierarchy of healing, each step builds on the foundation of the one before it.

I've used physical practices like yoga and dance, alongside herbs and nutrients, to help women stabilize, release emotions, and support this energy center. Intravenous nutrient therapy, visualizations, vitamins, and minerals can detoxify and clear the pain and emotional clutter stored in the body's cells, creating greater flow and vitality. Healing is interconnected—addressing one aspect inevitably supports the other.

Here, we focus on identifying your emotional code—the internal "software" running the show in your brain and body—by using the power of pause. I call this the **60-second rule for emotional freedom**. Whenever an emotion arises, remember: Emotions are messages trying to tell us something. Give yourself 60 seconds to fully feel it. If it's anger, close your eyes, take a full deep breath, and release it—maybe through a scream or a long, deep sigh.

You might wonder, *What if I'm in front of others or in a room full of people?* If it's not a safe space to express your emotion or take a time-out, you can still pause, close your eyes, and imagine yourself physically releasing it. For sadness, put your hands over your heart, breathe, and allow yourself to sit with the feeling and let the tears flow. If it's resentment, place one hand on your forehead and one over your heart and just notice where it lands in your body and what it feels like. This can be practiced with any emotion you are experiencing at any time. These 60 seconds of pause give you the space to engage with the ABCD rule of emotional bliss, which we'll explore next.

*A* is for accepting the emotion you are feeling, *B* for be curious about your reaction, *C* for creating an opportunity to learn more about yourself, and *D* for decoding the gift from this interaction. For example, by choosing **acceptance** over rejection, you create an opportunity to explore where the emotion is coming from and why it's surfacing in this moment. This process invites curiosity about yourself and your responses to different experiences. Below is a list of questions I encourage my patients to ask themselves as they work to accept and understand the deeper message their soul is trying to convey.

1. Is this emotion mine to experience, or does it belong to someone else?
2. What is the power of this emotion? For example, is my anger asking me to act on something? Is my sadness asking me to slow down and reconnect with myself?
3. Is there a pattern to this emotion? Does it show up at a certain time in my cycle?

4. Is this an emotion that has been with me for a long time? Did I have it as a child?
5. What makes me uncomfortable about this emotion?
6. How do I usually behave when I feel this emotion? Do I have habits that follow this emotion? What are they, and how do they serve or deplete my hormones and body?

This **curiosity** makes room for **learning**. It gives us permission to understand ourselves more deeply and recognize that the emotion is trying to help us decode a message that we may have been suppressing. This allows us to see the **gift** in that emotion—like the love that is being expressed in grief or the message of hormonal chaos in the irritability toward a partner.

To help women understand the connection between their hormones, emotions, and relationships, I use the following dialogue. It simplifies how past stresses and traumas have contributed to the emotional patterns they experience today, making the relationship between these elements easier to decode and learn from.

**Hormones/Emotions:** I'm burned-out and can't sleep and feel wired all day.

**Trauma/Stress Cycle:** I can't—if I slow down, I will have to face my wounds.

**Hormones/Emotions:** I feel angry and irritable and can't stand my husband, whom I love. Why can't I just pause and not react?

**Trauma/Stress Cycle:** I can't—if I do it feels like I'm giving my power away again and anger helps me feel some sense of power and control in the situation.

**Hormones/Emotions:** I'm feeling really depressed and wanting to isolate because I can't stand how I feel, how I look, and who I am.

**Trauma/Stress Cycle:** I was never made to feel like what I had to say was important and was criticized for being myself and speaking up, making me question my self-worth.

**Hormones/Emotions:** I'm feeling resentful, low energy, and have no desire for intimacy, and I overthink every decision.

**Trauma/Stress Cycle:** Love was conditional growing up and was withdrawn from me when I didn't behave as others wanted me to. I learned I can only receive it by putting others' needs first and overpleasing.

The more we learn about where the source of our emotional pattern is from, the easier it gets to understand the gift they have been all along. It is here we get to reflect from the learning what the gift we received from the experiences in our past was, and here is where we get to decide what we are ready to let go of to move forward so we are in the driver's seat, not our emotions.

I invite you now to take some time to write down the various emotions in your life that come up regularly and try to decode their story just as we have been decoding yours. Take the time to reflect on the questions listed before to help you uncover a new relationship to yourself!

## The Mental Level

When you master your mind, you gain the power to shape your world and manifest the life and health you desire. Our minds hold immense power—they can turn a day into one filled with joy and possibility or one consumed by sorrow and pain, depending on which part of the mind we let take charge. In yogic traditions, the mind is understood to have three aspects: the negative mind, which serves as a protector; the positive mind, which acts as an expander; and the neutral mind, which serves as the observer. It is from the neutral mind that we strive to make decisions and manifest our desires.

When we have and are experiencing stress, the mind's ability to discern and utilize the neutral mind is challenged by the emotions we are feeling in the experience. By strengthening the discernment in the mind, we take away the hold the emotions have on our state.

Both positive and negative minds love feedback loops. For example, when you have a habit that you know doesn't support your health, maybe it's drinking wine every evening, the negative mind assures you it's exactly what you need to protect your nervous system from the long, hard day you just had, and the positive mind assures you that you deserve it and reminds you of how relaxed you feel in the moment as the liquid hits your cells. Both thoughts and minds are then reinforced by the temporary relief you feel in the moment, removing any foresight into how you usually feel the next day after a restless sleep due to too much alcohol the night before. The only way to change this pattern or feedback loop is to utilize that neutral mind through practices such as meditation and mindful awareness.

When guiding women to build a healthier relationship with their mind, it becomes essential to address the third chakra—the solar plexus—which governs personal power, confidence, and mental clarity. This energy center is deeply connected to the mind's ability to process, discern, and make decisions. Mastering the solar plexus helps a woman tap into a wellspring of inner wisdom, allowing her to express herself with ease and self-assurance. With confidence comes the ability to trust the mind's capacity to distinguish between its different aspects and foresee the potential consequences of its choices. Mastering the mind, cultivating confidence, and sharpening discernment are key steps in breaking free from limiting beliefs and conditioned patterns, replacing them with ones that promote health and growth. Before exploring techniques to strengthen your connection with your mind, take a moment to reflect on what the mind means to you.

1. How would you define the mind and your relationship to it?
2. What beliefs do you hold about yourself? Beliefs around self-worth, around your identity, and who you are supposed to be. (It can be helpful to write "I am" statements.)
3. Out of those beliefs, which ones are true, which ones were given to you, and which ones did you create to protect yourself?
4. What does your mind tell you about your health? Is it always looking for what's wrong?

5. Do you feel scattered in your mind, if yes, does this get magnified in certain times of your cycle (or once you were in perimenopause or menopause)?
6. Are you easily distracted or need distraction when things feel hard?
7. Have you experienced the power of your mind before? Is there an example of a time when you consciously chose to think something different that changed the outcome of an experience?

There is immense power in a decision. I remember when I was struggling with anorexia, it took one shift in mindset to begin my healing journey. I decided that my resentment toward my family would no longer control my health or my future, and from that moment, I never looked back. What we focus on—whether it's a belief, mindset, or habit—gains energy and power, shaping our reality. By focusing on what supports our healing and vitality, we can transform our experience into one of health and growth. The physical changes caused by fluctuating hormones are real, but without a shift in mindset, healing can only go so far. Change your mind, and you'll change your hormones. Change your emotions, and you'll transform your relationships.

Here are a few mantras and affirmations that can help you shift from one mind state to another when you are feeling stuck or overwhelmed.

- *Satnam*—Truth is my identity, and in oneness I connect.
- I am courageous and I am decisive.
- *Waheguru*—I am in awe of myself and the light within that can guide me from dark to light.
- I get to choose.
- *Nirbhau; nirvair*—Without fear; without hate

I encourage you to choose one of the mantras above and meditate on it for a few minutes each day, repeating it out loud with intention. Approach this practice with the goal of shifting a belief, and after 40 days, revisit your "I am" statements and beliefs about your identity. You may be surprised by how much clarity emerges as you let go of thoughts and beliefs that were never truly yours. Mastering your mind is about mastering the art of discernment—the ability to hear beyond the noise and see through the fog of old patterns and limiting beliefs. This clarity gives you the courage to view your relationship with yourself and others with a fresh, empowered perspective.

## The Relational Level

Healing can often feel like a lonely journey, but sharing our joys and pains with others opens the door to connection, which is vital for true healing. The quality of our relationships directly reflects the level of fulfillment we feel in our lives. Loneliness, on the other hand, can lead to depression, and its impact extends to our physical health as much as our mental well-being. When hormones feel chaotic, it becomes challenging to articulate the inner turmoil a woman may feel in both body and mind. Women in perimenopause and menopause often experience a drop in estrogen that drives them toward isolation, even if they don't fully understand why. The changes in their bodies can feel overwhelming and difficult to explain—like switching from a parka to a tank top within moments, flushed and disoriented. Yet, it is precisely through connection and feeling safe in our relationships that healing becomes possible. Going to bed with a sense of peace and contentment in our connections allows the body to relax and surrender to restful sleep. In contrast, relational conflict keeps the brain on high alert, preventing the nervous system from trusting and letting go, which blocks your hormones from fully healing.

*Interpersonal synchronization* refers to the phenomenon where our physiological rhythms, such as breathing patterns and heart rates, align with those of the people we spend time with, particularly romantic partners. Studies show that when you are with your partner, your bodies' rhythms can literally sync up. This also means that when you're feeling stressed or out of balance due to hormonal changes, your partner may be experiencing similar effects.

A 2017 study demonstrated the power of this connection: Empathetic partners who held their loved one's hand during moments of pain helped reduce that pain significantly. The more empathy the partner showed, the less pain was felt. This is largely due to the rise in oxytocin, the "bonding hormone," which is released when we feel connected to others.

In the Hierarchy of Hormonal Healing, fostering connection plays a vital role in healing the relational piece. This process is energetically linked to the fourth chakra—the heart center. When we lead with the heart, we honor our innate wisdom and prioritize love over fear or frustration. This heart-led state fosters connection and healing. However, when we distance our hearts from others, our emotions can take over, making it harder to pause and reflect before reacting. Practicing the 60 seconds to emotional freedom, a skill we learned earlier in the chapter, can help bring us back to the heart's wisdom, ensuring we respond with love rather than letting emotions control us.

Your relationships are your best teachers in the school of you. Each significant relationship in your life gives you an opportunity to unlearn old patterns that hurt you and learn more about your truth. Your physical, emotional, and mental health in the hierarchy influence the health of your relationships just as much as the dynamics of your relationship impact them. This invites us to ask the question, what is the source of stress in any relationship?

If we feel healthy and clear in our body and mind, would that help us communicate clearly and have discernment in our relationships? Or are we reliant on the relationship to create health in our body and mind?

Numerous studies have shown that healthy social relationships contribute to better health outcomes and greater resilience in coping with stress. While I wholeheartedly agree with these findings, I've also observed that it's challenging to bring the right energy and clarity into relationships when your body and mind feel fatigued, cluttered, or unwell. Many of my patients have shared how their relationships transformed after healing their hormones and detoxifying their bodies and minds. When you care for your hormones, you naturally nurture your relationships. Similarly, when your relationships bring you joy, connection, and fulfillment, your physical and mental health improves significantly.

One activity I encourage all my patients to practice when working on their relationship with themselves and their heart is creating a Joy List. This is a list of activities, connections, and habits that bring you joy. Place it somewhere you'll see it daily and commit to choosing one thing from the list every day. This practice helps you stay connected to yourself, which in turn gives you the energy and capacity to connect meaningfully with others.

When you make a habit of carving out time for yourself, you create space to invite others into your joy-filled activities. These shared experiences foster connection and trigger oxytocin surges, reinforcing the joy you rightfully deserve. Research on happiness suggests that we may have a genetically determined "happiness set point." However, after learning about the influence of our environment, choices, and hormones on our emotions, it's clear to me that we hold the power to shift that set point toward greater joy in all aspects of life, especially in our relationships.

I recall observing how my mom would interact with my dad during small, everyday moments. Their relationship was always loving, but over time, my mom began expressing her voice more often through irritation and agitation. Reflecting now, I recognize that this shift began when she entered early menopause. Sometimes, I catch myself reacting to my husband in similar ways during certain points in my cycle. At first, I feel frustrated for not pausing in the moment, but then I remind myself that while my genetic makeup may have set a default, I have the power to choose differently. That realization is true empowerment and freedom: knowing that we always have a choice in how we show up, especially in our relationships, when we prioritize the most vital relationship of all—our relationship with ourselves.

Below, I've outlined what I believe are the essential ingredients for creating healthy, joyful relationships. These elements not only amplify joy in our personal lives but also ripple outward, spreading joy into the world.

## The Soul Level

In the shamanic medicine wheel, there is a practice where the practitioner helps the client bring pieces of her soul back that may have been scattered because of various stressors and trauma, helping her to feel whole again. This movement up the Hierarchy of Hormonal Healing does just that. It allows us to gather the pieces to be able to remember the wholeness we are and have always been. I lost a large piece of me as a child in that room where I was sexually molested. I lost my voice and trust in the world. I spent most of my adult life thinking I had nothing important to say and that it is too dangerous to speak, so for years I kept my thoughts to myself and was always scared to speak up, whether in a classroom or around the dinner table. I felt the safest in the shadows, just observing life around me, but my soul had other plans all along.

I once heard someone say that one of the greatest pains is when your outer world doesn't align with the potential you feel inside. For years, I carried that pain, a quiet ache that lingered until I finally found my voice. I began saying no, establishing the boundaries I so desperately needed, and transforming the relationships that no longer served me. I started speaking my truth. That's when my healing truly began, and for the first time, I could hear the gentle whispers of my soul. None of this would have been possible, though, without first clearing the clutter—physically, emotionally, mentally, and within my relationships.

When you reach this stage of healing, everything starts to align and make sense. You are no longer deceived by the maya, the illusion that once veiled your eyes and heart. Instead, you're deeply attuned to your inner knowing and connection to the source, making it nearly impossible for anything to cloud your vision. And if it does, you can quickly course correct. This stage involves healing the fifth, sixth, and seventh chakras—your voice, intuition, and universal connection—bringing them into harmony. When these centers are nurtured, you feel expansive, abundant, and

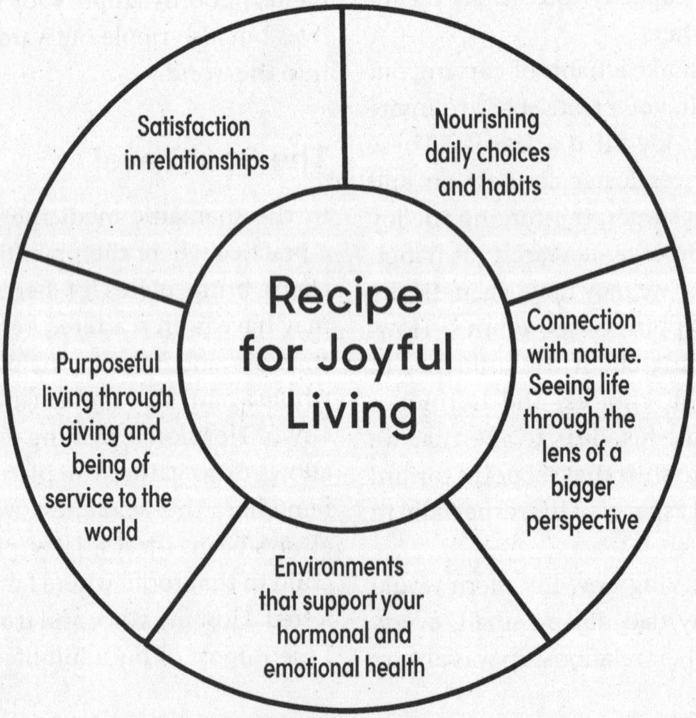

energized. You tap into the concept of *ek*, the oneness and unity between your physical, emotional, and spiritual selves. Practices like meditation and specific mantras help anchor you in this state, as their vibrational frequencies heal your cells at a deep level. Even something as simple as humming can deliver this healing energy, bringing balance and vitality to your entire being.

Most of the exercises and strategies at this level of healing are designed to enhance your vagal tone and autonomic flexibility—your ability to adapt to the world around you with awareness and a sense of peace. These practices essentially support the parasympathetic nervous system, helping you rest, digest, and heal through activation of your vagus nerve, the longest nerve in your body. By doing so, you become more open to hearing the true narrator of your story: your soul. Research has shown a strong link between higher vagal tone and positive emotions, improved social connections, and better physical outcomes. Additionally, studies indicate that infants born to mothers who experienced anger, depression, or anxiety during pregnancy often have lower vagal tone, which can impact their emotional and behavioral regulation. Strengthening your vagal tone is essential for hormonal healing. Fortunately, there are specific habits and practices you can incorporate into your daily life to support and improve it.

One of my favorite mantra and breathing exercises to help me connect with my soul and ease my hormonal discomforts and anxieties is *So hum.*

*Sit quietly in a comfortable position and notice your breath. As you witness your inhale and exhale, begin to feel into its rhythm and into its depth. Place one hand on your forehead and another on your heart. As you inhale, begin to chant* So, *meaning the divine and your connection to it, and on the exhale as you let it all go,* Hum, *meaning I and the ego self. Practice this for a few minutes and watch the anxieties, worries, and discomforts dissolve as you release the hold on what was to invite what is meant to be, a state of ease and healing.*

Moving through the Hierarchy of Hormonal Healing takes courage, consistency, and commitment. If you allow yourself to access those three potentials inside of you, there is nothing or no one that can hold you back from living your best life, no matter what age and no matter what stage you are in, in your hormonal journey.

Now that you've explored the concept of Hormonal Hierarchy and how each hormone plays a distinct role in your overall well-being, the next step is to understand **your unique hormonal identity**. Just like no two stories are the same, no two hormone patterns are exactly alike. In the next chapter, you'll begin to identify the dominant energies within your hormonal landscape—your personal chemistry, your tendencies, and how they influence your mood, energy, and relationships. With this understanding, you'll be able to apply the principles of Hormonal Hierarchy in a way that's tailored to *you*—bringing clarity to your symptoms and guiding you toward more aligned healing choices.

| RITUAL/HABIT/ LIFESTYLE | OPTIONS | WHY |
|---|---|---|
| Movement | Yoga | Can improve vagal tone through raising heart rate variability and supporting the parasympathetic nervous system and reducing levels of stress |
| Breathwork | Long, deep diaphragmatic breathing<br>Ujjayi and Brahmari Breath | Downregulates the sympathetic nervous system while inducing relaxation in body and mind |
| Cold exposure | Ending your shower with 30 seconds of cold water against your body, starting with your forehead | Can regulate the fight-or-flight response |
| Humming, gargling, and chanting | Mantras or any good song that gets you in a joyful mood | The vagus nerve runs through the larynx and pharynx in your throat, so these practices create a vibration, activating the nerve. |
| Meditation | Visualization<br>Walking meditation in nature<br>Silent meditation on a concept, a word, an affirmation | Eases the mind and relaxes the nervous system, allowing the vagal tone to be stimulated |
| Power of touch | Massage therapy, especially with warming oils like sesame oil, for your nervous system; a little sesame oil on the soles of your feet before bed can help your nervous system relax throughout the night | Decreases sympathetic response in the body, creating a safe and nurturing experience in your body |
| Probiotics | *Lactobacillus rhamnosus*<br>*Bifidobacterium longum* | *Lactobacillus* helps activate GABA, a calming neurotransmitter<br>*Bifidobacterium* has anxiolytic effects and supports the gut-brain connection |
| Connection | Socializing and creating space for your joy list | Connecting with others and consciously choosing joy helps relax your nervous system. |
| Grounding | Barefoot in nature<br>Time away from technology<br>Red light therapy to counteract excessive blue light exposure | Nature helps your vagus nerve get back into its intended rhythm, because there is so much in our lives that takes us out of that rhythm, like blue light from screens. |

CHAPTER 8

# Finding Your Hormonal Identity

Every woman has a unique hormonal fingerprint—a blend of chemistry, rhythm, and experience that shapes how she feels, thinks, and responds to the world. In this chapter, you'll begin uncovering your **hormonal identity** so you can better understand the patterns that drive your emotions, energy, and cycles—and learn how to work with them, not against them.

When self-discovery begins, we start to uncover who we are meant to be, whom we need to let go of, and the wise woman we have always been. This awakening allows us to step into a state of adaptability, enabling us to navigate the vast array of stressors life throws our way—whether they come from environmental toxins, emotional turmoil, or negative thought patterns. Adaptability is a key tool in managing the physical, mental, and emotional stressors that often manifest as symptoms in the body and disrupt hormonal balance. When we cultivate this resilience, we empower our body to process and respond to stress more effectively, reducing its impact on our nervous system, digestion, and reproductive health. By becoming adaptable, we give our body the space to restore harmony, stabilize our hormones, and prevent chronic stress from becoming the root cause of imbalance.

Developing the ability to adapt physically, mentally, and emotionally fosters resilience and vitality, diminishing the fear of the uncontrollable—whether it's the food at a holiday party, the mold in your office building, or the behavior of a parent. While the body and mind instinctively resist the unknown, as we've explored earlier, it's often this fear that prevents us from embracing transformative changes, taking bold steps, or fully committing to the healing journey.

When the mind and body experience a sense of adaptability, they release the grip of fear and emotion, creating a profound sense of trust and security. For example, learning to adapt by shifting food habits—like reducing inflammatory foods or incorporating more nutrient-dense meals—can ease digestive discomfort, balance hormones, and build trust in your body's ability to heal. Similarly, practicing mindfulness or breathwork to navigate emotional triggers helps you stay grounded, reducing the stress response that might otherwise spiral into anxiety or physical symptoms like tension headaches or fatigue. These small, adaptive changes signal to your body and mind that they are safe, fostering a healing environment where balance and resilience can flourish.

The ADAPT formula provides a framework for understanding how to achieve this lasting transformation. Before diving into the formula, take a moment to reflect and answer the following questions to prepare yourself for breaking old cycles for good.

1. Where have you been sourcing your story from? For example, from your culture, family, a past experience?
2. How has this story shaped how you see the world? For example, do you feel the need to be in control to feel safe? Or do you feel like you need to please others to feel loved?
3. Who has become your narrator? Whose voice or voices have you been hearing in your mind all these years?
4. Where do you feel stuck in the following categories?
5. Take a moment to draw a picture of a symbol, an archetype, an animal, anything that you feel represents a state of health and freedom. This image can act as an anchor and reminder of where you are going and where you really want to be. (I like to imagine myself as Wonder Woman on a mission to change the way women see their hormones, accompanied by a wolf. I tell you, it works to get me out my funk every time!)

| Health | Purpose |
|---|---|
| | |
| **Spirituality** | **Relationships** |
| | |

## The HER Method: ADAPT

There are seasons to everything. First, the leaves fall from the trees, then the ground hardens under winter's blanket, followed by the fresh vibrance of spring, with birds chirping and flowers blooming, before the heat of summer takes over. Nature moves through constant, inevitable change. It doesn't resist, because this cycle is essential for growth. Instead, it adapts. Similarly, our ability to adapt to our environment shapes the outcomes of our journey.

In one scenario, adaptation arises from a need for survival. When the environment feels unsafe, you learn to suppress your feelings, shift your identity, and adjust how you navigate your days to cope and protect yourself. In another, adaptation is intentional—a course correction driven by a desire to heal, grow, and restore balance after environmental disruptors have caused chaos.

It's through this intentional adaptation that your hormones can regain harmony, transmitting clear signals from one cell to the next. Understanding how to embrace this process allows you to heal the wounds of survival-based adaptations and shift into a space of thriving. It is the bridge that carries you from enduring life's challenges to flourishing in its possibilities. Here I use the word *ADAPT* to describe the steps that you will take in the coming chapters to heal and transform your health and your story. *A* for awareness, *D* for discernment, *A* for action, *P* for pattern disruption, and finally *T* for transformation.

## The Power of Awareness

Awareness. Awareness of self, your surroundings, your story, your triggers, and anything and everything that could cause disruption and chaos in your inner world. The ability to become self-aware creates personal power. You become the controller and commander of the world around you instead of the other way around. Self-awareness allows you to see where you are stuck in your habits, your story, and your beliefs that are influencing how you feel in your body.

There's a well-known story about a Zen master and his student. The student visits the master seeking wisdom, but as the master speaks, the student repeatedly interrupts, eager to share his own beliefs and ideas. After a while, the master begins pouring tea into the student's cup. Even when the cup overflows, the master continues pouring. Alarmed, the student exclaims, "Why don't you stop? The cup is already full!"

The master calmly replies, "When your mind is full of your own ideas and assumptions, there's no room for new knowledge or growth."

This story illustrates the importance of releasing rigidity, habits, and patterns that may keep us stuck in cycles of discomfort and symptoms. When our "cup" is filled to the brim with the noise of daily life and the struggle to simply get by, it's difficult to envision change or create space for something new. We often cling to the same routines, environments, and habits that perpetuate our challenges.

However, true transformation begins when we recognize that what we've been doing isn't working and cultivate curiosity about the choices that keep us stuck. Self-awareness is the key to unlocking this freedom. It's not about self-blame but about becoming self-curious—examining our patterns, understanding our needs, and making space for growth. When we clear our "cup," we can finally get to know the real, thriving version of ourselves.

## The Power of Discernment

Discernment is essential for distinguishing what is real from the illusions (maya) that cloud our lives. Without it, we remain stuck in confusion, unsure which path to take. Only through the journey of self-knowledge and self-mastery can we fully grasp the reality we're living in. Without discernment, the soul's whispers are drowned out by the noise of the life we think we should be living. It becomes difficult to tell whether our reactions—like frustration toward a partner—stem from hormonal shifts or require deeper exploration. We may fail to recognize if the food we eat or the environments we frequent are harming or helping our health. For years, we might follow family traditions like consuming inflammatory foods without realizing the toll they take on our hormones, brain, and gut health. Some powerful questions that I seed for my patients when stepping into discernment are:

"Will this choice nourish me or deplete me?"

"Will my future self thank me for this decision, or will she be faced with regret?"

"Is the voice that is asking for this my own, or is it my old narrator?"

"Will this help build my triangle of empowerment or break it down?"

These are simple questions but can create profound opportunity toward self-knowledge.

## The Power of Action

Returning to the discussion about the cells in your body—nothing happens without decisive action between one cell and the next. Energy cannot be created, movement cannot occur, detoxification cannot take place, and hormonal messages cannot be relayed without a commitment to act. At the cellular level, this is driven by the action potential, a spike or impulse of electrical activity that allows cells to communicate. Without it, progress halts. Now consider what this means for you: What kind of impulse or catalyst would inspire you to take decisive action in your life?

From my own experience and what I've witnessed in others, it begins with an unshakable belief in the importance of the next step. When we deeply understand why certain actions—such as taking specific herbs, eliminating certain foods, or starting hormone therapy—are necessary, it becomes easier to take the right steps to build healthy habits. Repeating those actions consistently rewires the brain, forming new circuits and patterns. Eventually, what once felt unfamiliar becomes second nature.

Patients often share how they no longer crave sugary foods, react with anger, or prioritize others' needs over their own. Instead, they feel empowered to take the actions that truly support their health and well-being. This conscious shift paves the way for a life filled with meaning, purpose, and freedom as you take matters into your own hands and act from your own intentions toward health.

## The Power of Pattern Disruption

Do you ever find yourself going through the motions of your day without fully realizing how much you've done? You've worked all day, picked up the kids, driven them to their activities, made dinner, and now you're finally sitting on the couch, ready for bed. It feels like the day flew by in a blink, with you operating on autopilot, moving through your daily routine. This external experience mirrors your internal world, which also runs on its historical patterns unless you consciously intervene. In the early stages of change, your brain may resist because it craves comfort and familiarity.

For some, the more direct, yang approach—cutting things out completely or diving straight into something new—is the best way to disrupt old patterns. For others, a softer, yin approach, like repeating affirmations or using a mantra, can gently shift the narrative. Simple tools for disrupting patterns include asking the reflective questions mentioned earlier, walking around the perimeter of the grocery store instead of through the aisles of processed foods, or making small daily changes to your routine. For example, instead of diving into work right away, take a walk around the block first to clear your mind. These small acts of disruption create a state change, offering you the freedom to consciously choose how you move through your day and be fully present in each moment.

## The Power of Transformation

I once heard a friend say, "Nature is my religion," and I loved that. To me, any spiritual practice is one that transforms our personal wants and desires into something that serves not just us, but everyone. It's a pathway to purpose. When I observe nature—especially through the lens of the medicine wheel—I feel a deep responsibility to be an earth keeper, someone who recognizes the gifts Mother Nature offers and strives to honor her in the best way possible. Nature is a constant force of transformation, always in her purpose, and that same force resides within each of us.

When we feel stuck in our symptoms or stories, it may seem impossible to imagine transformation. But when we cultivate awareness, practice discernment, take intentional action, and disrupt the patterns that keep us stagnant, nothing can stand in the way of our growth. The vibrant, healed version of yourself that you envision becomes a reality—not through choices imposed on you, but through the ones you consciously make. Transformation becomes possible when we let go of rigidity and remain curious, open to change. By releasing rigid habits and patterns, we free ourselves from suffering in both body and mind, inviting flow and ease into our lives.

You are no longer a victim of your past stories, traumas, or routines. Instead, you are empowered by the knowledge that you can create change and that you are worthy of transformation. As you evolve, so do your relationships and the world around you.

## HER Hormonal Identity

The Hormonal Hierarchy offers a framework of priorities, one that I've found essential in my practice. This structure helps disrupt the cycle of hormonal identities many of us unconsciously cling to. These identities shape how we show up in the world, how we carry our stresses, and how those stresses manifest as symptoms in the body. When you've lived a certain way for so long, it's difficult to recognize patterns that others might easily see. It's like the saying "the fish are the last to discover the water," because they've been swimming in it their entire lives—they know nothing else.

The identities we hold, the roles we play, and the masks we wear become what we believe to be our truth. To uncover the reality beyond these layers requires introspection, courage, and commitment. The symptoms you experience are your body's way of signaling the toll of moving through these identity cycles, often adopted for survival. Whether these patterns were mirrored for you or born out of necessity, the first step to breaking free is acknowledging the physical

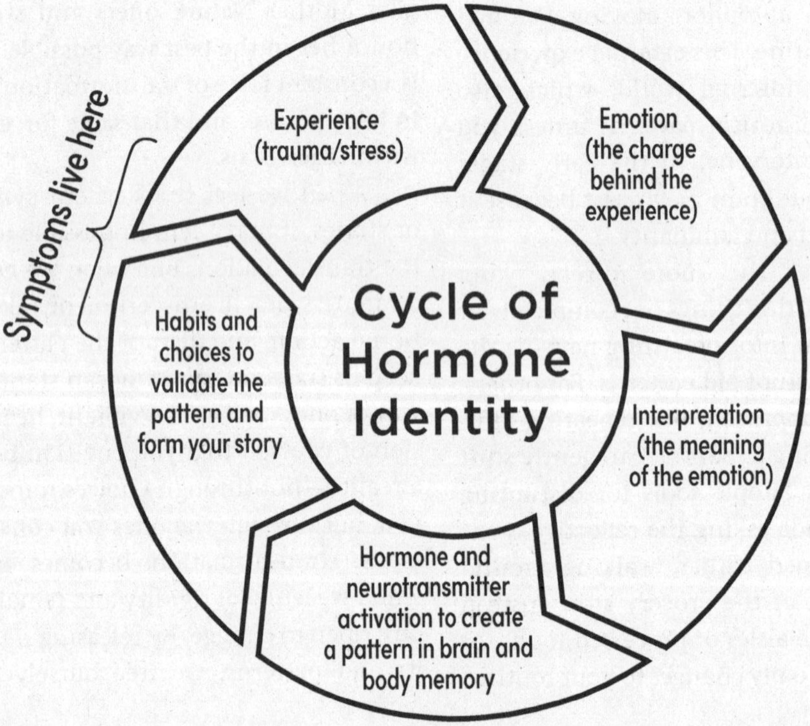

toll they've taken. From there, applying the ADAPT formula can guide you in dismantling the cycle and creating lasting change.

The body speaks through its symptoms, helping us uncover the language of our hormonal identity. By examining your current hormonal identity and the symptoms you're experiencing, we can identify the next essential steps for healing. These identities are often reinforced by habitual lifestyle choices. Once you understand the link between these choices and the autopilot behaviors driving them, it becomes much easier to create change.

Take, for example, the common "evening wine and dine" ritual many women fall into. It might start as a way for a woman to unwind after a long, stressful day—whether at work, with the kids, or simply from feeling overwhelmed. The initial trigger is stress, which sends a signal that something is needed to shift her state. That first sip of wine provides warmth and relaxation, calming her nervous system. Over time, the ritual takes on significant meaning: It becomes her reward for surviving the day, a moment of self-care. Initially, her hormones might respond positively, but as time goes on, the ritual begins to disrupt her melatonin production, impairing sleep quality. Despite the negative effects, the thought of giving up this routine creates stress, because it feels like the only thing that's just for her.

Change often becomes possible only when our body reaches a state of depletion, manifesting in symptoms like hot flashes, night sweats, insomnia, or weight gain. This is the turning point—a clear signal that it's time to break the cycle and restore balance.

I have grouped three identities that I feel many of us can relate to. Some may fall into all three, while others might feel like they are anchored in one. By completing the Hormone Identity Quiz on the pages ahead, you can get a sense of where to start with your healing, and in the coming chapters, we will break each archetype down and give you protocols and support for each.

As you complete the quiz, for each question, mark 0 for Never, 1 for Sometimes, and 2 for Always. The identity with the highest score likely reflects your dominant hormonal identity at this moment. While you may resonate with aspects of multiple identities, identifying your primary one can provide valuable insights into your body's current needs and the treatment that will best support you. The descriptions that follow outline some key traits associated with these identities. This quiz is not intended to serve as a comprehensive diagnostic tool but rather as a guide to help you understand the link between the identity you've created and its impact on your hormonal health. By recognizing the choices this identity makes to cope with life's stressors, you gain the power to rewrite your story and unravel your hormonal blueprint.

## Identity #1

1. Do you feel like you are rushing from one task to the next?
2. Do you feel like you need to be in charge or have a sense of control in most experiences?
3. Did you grow up feeling you only received love if you performed as you parents needed you to?
4. Do you compare your successes to other people's successes?
5. Do you have sleep disturbances?
6. Do you have an afternoon slump of energy and need coffee or other stimulants to pick you up?
7. Do you feel anxious?
8. Do you suffer from mood changes before your period?
9. Do you have pain in your body or menstrual cramps?
10. Do you suffer from night sweats?
11. Do you deal with brain fog?
12. Do you tend to gain weight around your abdomen?
13. Do you thrive on having a high-paced life?
14. Is your libido low?
15. Do you feel agitated or irritated often?

## Identity #2

1. Do you tend to put others' needs before your needs?
2. Do you tend to feel that your opinion does not matter or feel like you don't have anything important to say?
3. Do you tend to shy away from being seen, either at work or at home or in a crowd?
4. Do you feel like you need to say yes to everything and everyone, no matter the cost to your health?
5. Do you feel you crash in the evening?
6. Do you have low energy?
7. Do you have cold hands and feet?
8. Is your hair thinning or falling out?
9. Has anyone in your family had a cancer diagnosis?
10. Do you feel alone and isolated?
11. Do you feel easily flustered, especially when you don't know how to do something?
12. Do you have digestive issues, bloating, diarrhea, or constipation?
13. Does your inner voice criticize you often?
14. Do you feel that no matter what you do, or what you have, that it just isn't enough?
15. Do you see the world from a glass-half-empty perspective?

## Identity #3

1. Do you feel like you need to keep up an image of perfection for others?
2. Have you tried all the different diets and still can't seem to find the right one for you?
3. Do you have heavy bleeds?
4. Do you have fibrocystic breasts?
5. Do you get sick and then find your recovery period to be long?
6. Is commitment hard for you? Whether to a relationship or a nutrition plan?
7. Do you have skin blemishes?
8. Do you ignore shadow emotions like anger?
9. Do you struggle with feeling enough?
10. Do you have hot flashes?
11. Have you ever felt stuck in your life?
12. Do you have vaginal dryness?
13. Do you have cravings for sweets?
14. Do you often suffer from headaches or migraines right before your period?
15. Do you feel hypoglycemic?

Once you've answered the questions, count how many points you have in the responses you have for each identity. The identity with the highest score likely represents the one you're navigating at this moment. These identities can shift depending on the season of life you're in and may not reflect your true essence but rather a learned or adaptive way of coping with current circumstances. Next, you'll find brief descriptions of each identity and insights into how they may influence your day-to-day life.

## Identity #1: The Anxious Overachiever

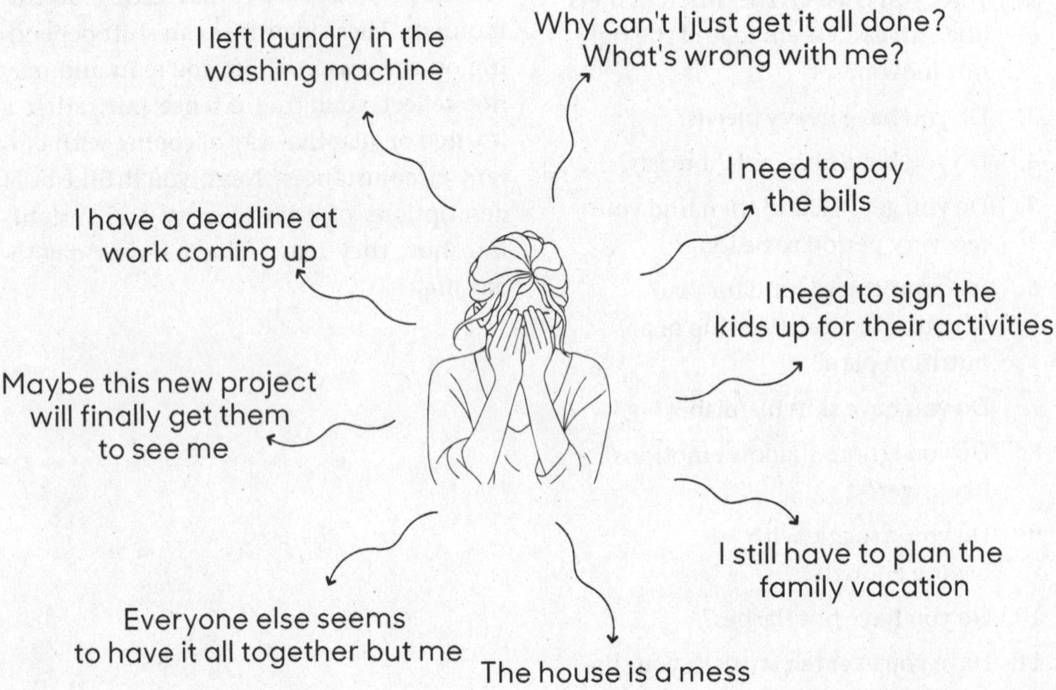


This identity often carries an intensity that leaves her constantly on edge, looking disheveled, and overwhelmed by the stress weighing her down. She feels a deep need to prove herself, carrying an old story from her past that fuels her drive. Relaxation feels impossible as she moves through her days, trying to fit everything in. Despite her many successes, she struggles to see the positives, especially within herself, and is her own harshest critic. Self-doubt lingers as an ever-present companion. Overwhelmed by responsibilities and unresolved symptoms, she has no time to prioritize her health. Her chronic stress has led to stubborn belly fat, no matter the diet, along with anxiety, bouts of depression, irregular periods, and debilitating PMS. She's perpetually exhausted, leaving little to no room for intimacy, even though she deeply loves her partner. Women in this state often push themselves until their body finally forces them to pause, screaming for attention and healing.

The primary focus of her healing must be her nervous system. Without calming her stress response, no other aspect of her health will improve. In tandem with identifying which hormones need support, it is crucial to help her transition from a constant fight-or-flight state into a more relaxed and balanced state. This shift is essential for her overall healing and well-being.

Let me share a story about this identity. I had a patient, Jessica, a 45-year-old woman with a high-paced job and two children. From the outside, she seemed like someone who had it all together—highly organized and capable of managing everything. But as we spoke, she revealed the overwhelming guilt she carried every day. She felt guilty about her kids while she was at work and guilty about work when she was with her kids. She had set an impossible standard for herself: parenting as if she didn't have a job and working as if she didn't have a family.

Years of this internal battle finally took a toll on her physical and mental health. Her periods had become irregular; she struggled with insomnia, constant brain fog, and a lack of libido, and relied on coffee just to make it through the day. When we dove deeper into her story, she shared that as a child, she often had to walk on eggshells around her mother, unsure of what mood she would encounter. Her coping mechanism had been to stay quiet, keep her head down and her needs to herself, and meet expectations as a high achiever to maintain peace.

It became clear that to help her, we needed to first address her nervous system and disrupt the pattern of stress. Over the next few months, we worked on implementing habits and support to ease the stress reaction in her body to give her a taste of what it felt like to feel grounded and steady. As her nervous system began to regulate with new daily habits from different food choices to supplements and hormones, she was ready to go deeper into the healing process. She noticed that even small shifts in her energy had a profound effect on her family dynamics—her kids and husband seemed calmer, and their interactions were easier.

She began communicating more openly and even started asking for help—one of the hardest things for her to do. She also realized how deeply attached she had been to her identity as the one who always had to manage it all. While the calmness initially felt foreign and even uncomfortable, she could see the positive changes in her body and relationships. This progress motivated her to continue moving forward with her health plan.

## Identity #2: The Silent Struggler

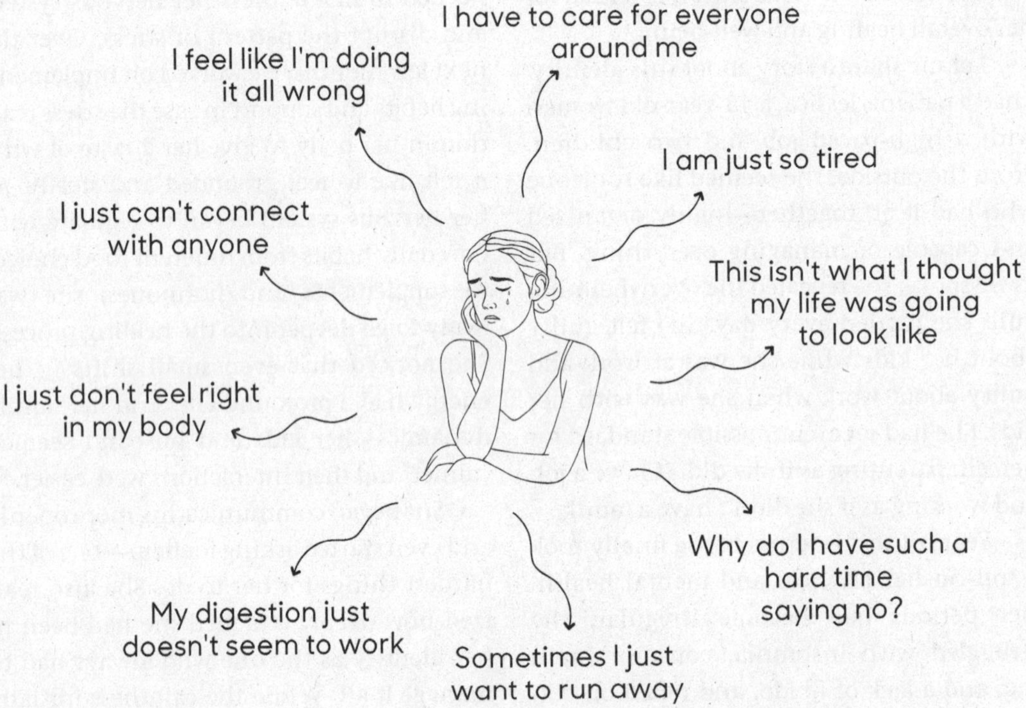


This identity silently carries the weight of the world while serving as the anchor for everyone around her. She is the person others rely on, and she often finds her sense of purpose and significance in her role as the caregiver. However, this comes at a cost—leaving her feeling depleted and harboring silent resentment.

When anger and resentment build due to her difficulty in speaking her truth, her immune and hormonal systems often bear the burden. Chronic physical and emotional pain can take hold. For her, the healing journey begins with nourishment—physically, emotionally, and mentally.

The process of unlearning and releasing this deeply ingrained identity will take time, but the first step is to replenish and nurture her body. By focusing on building her physical strength, supporting her hormones, and bolstering her immune system, she can begin to gather the resilience needed to speak her truth and share her authentic self with the world.

Barb is a patient I've had the privilege of working with for years. She started seeing me in her early 20s, and I've had the joy of watching her grow into her power as a woman. With her sweet demeanor, she's loved by everyone around her. When she first came to me, she was dealing with chronic vaginal infections, skin issues, chronic fatigue, bloating, and irregular periods. Her body was clearly depleted and crying out for help.

We began by testing her hormones, running a food sensitivity test, and checking for thyroid antibodies. Sure enough, she was diagnosed with Hashimoto's thyroiditis, an autoimmune condition of the thyroid, along with numerous food sensitivities and significant stress from school, family, and a relationship.

As we unpacked her story, it became clear that the first priority was to rebuild her energy and vitality before diving into deeper treatments. Hashimoto's often stems from toxicity in the body, so while detoxing was a long-term goal, we needed to give her system reserves to work with first. What became really clear for her through her healing was that she had a really hard time saying no to others. By constantly saying yes to others, she was saying no to herself and her needs. After much self-reflection, yoga, and using her voice—even in small moments like when the waiter brought her the wrong meal, or when someone cut in front of her in line—she was able to find the courage to speak up for what she needs and change her physical health. We implemented an IV nutrition protocol, gut and adrenal support, and bioidentical hormones to give her a much-needed physical boost as she redefined her relationships and was beginning to understand what she wanted to manifest in her life.

Within a few weeks, she began to feel better, and we were able to transition into a detox phase. Gradually, her cycle regulated, her immune system strengthened, and although she's still on her health journey, it's evident how empowered she feels—even when new challenges arise. She has learned to listen to her body and respond with the care it needs. I'm inspired by her journey and her understanding that her body will always reflect the environment she creates for it, whether influenced by age, stress, or life itself.

## Identity #3: The Perfectionist with a Price

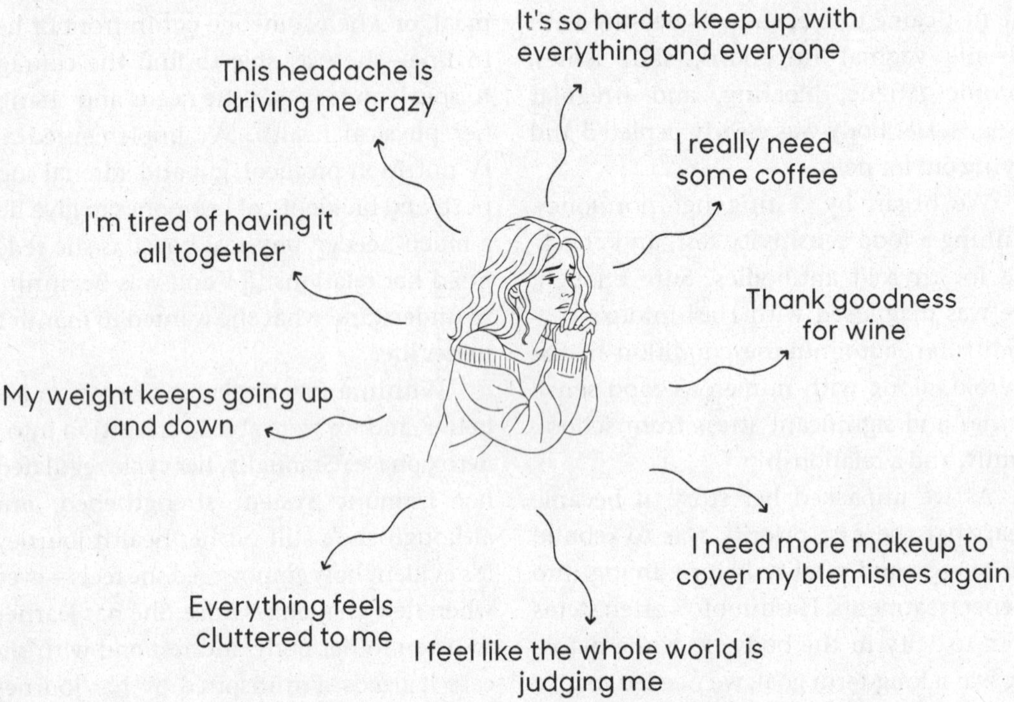
It's so hard to keep up with everything and everyone
This headache is driving me crazy
I really need some coffee
I'm tired of having it all together
Thank goodness for wine
My weight keeps going up and down
I need more makeup to cover my blemishes again
Everything feels cluttered to me
I feel like the whole world is judging me

On the outside, everything appears immaculate, but inside, she's in turmoil. She's tried it all—the diets, the exercise routines—but still finds herself stuck, questioning everything she does and everyone she connects with. Relationships are difficult. Trusting others is even harder. Her body and mind are burdened with toxins, both chemical and emotional, and she leans on vices like coffee, wine, and food to get through the discomfort of her façade and the masks she wears. She's trying her best, desperately working to change, yet finds herself falling back into old patterns, focused on maintaining the outward appearance of perfection.

If everything isn't perfect, she fears it will all fall apart. In her past, imperfection led to love being withheld, and now she pours herself into everything, yet when the veil of perfection slips even slightly, fear sets in, and she withdraws before any hurt can reach her. Her body feels trapped, stuck in this cycle.

The priority in her healing is to create more flexibility and flow—both physically and emotionally. Detoxing her body, mind, and emotions will help clear the internal clutter, allowing her to show up in the world unveiled, not from a place of fear but with confidence and self-love.

A 37-year-old woman, Samantha, came to me after experiencing multiple miscarriages. She cried as she shared her sorrow, guilt, and shame over what her body and her relationship were going through. She had been diagnosed with PCOS and was suspected to have endometriosis. It was clear she was carrying immense emotional pain and felt utterly alone. I talked with her about the potential causes behind her miscarriages and explained what a healthy environment in the reproductive system looks like, highlighting the significant role stress can play. As she began to understand these factors, she felt not only heard but also hopeful, realizing that she wasn't broken and that other solutions were possible.

Testing revealed she was in an estrogen-dominant state and faced multiple environmental challenges, including a poor diet, a mold-filled office, and chronic emotional stress. Our immediate priority was to clear her external and internal environments. We removed obstacles such as genetically modified foods, processed items, and unhealthy fats while addressing the mold issue in her home office.

After undergoing a thorough six-month detox, she felt healthier than ever. During this time, we also incorporated bioidentical progesterone, hormone-supporting herbs, nutrients to enhance mitochondrial function, IV therapy, and a consistent practice of self-care and self-love. Today, she's a happy mother of two, and her journey of overcoming the narrative she once believed has given her courage in many other areas of her life.

These identities, as necessary as they may have been, can hold us back from truly knowing ourselves and understanding what we need to heal. Often, we embody aspects of multiple identities. By identifying which personality or identity is currently dominant in your life, you can prioritize your healing and begin peeling back the layers to reveal your true self.

Navigating the Hormonal Hierarchy and uncovering your hormonal identity provides you with the tools to unlearn old habits and establish new ones that promote balance and well-being on every level. Letting go of an identity isn't always easy. These identities have served as a framework for how we operate in the world, offering a sense of familiarity and safety. To release what we know can trigger fear and doubt. However, by understanding yourself and how these identities were formed, it becomes easier to let go of what no longer serves you and step into the vibrant life you deserve.

## Taking Up Space

Regardless of which identity resonates with you or feels most present in this season of your life, one universal truth remains: Every identity has a right to take up space, and this is something we, as women, must learn to embrace. Each identity has its own set of gifts. These identities have not been working against you—they've been working for you, even if you've unknowingly been adopting habits or carrying stories that have created disharmony in your body. By recognizing the duality within each identity, we can honor their strengths while healing the parts causing chaos. The stressed-out overachiever is someone who can always get the job done. The caretaker is the dependable rock others turn to. The perfectionist is a mirror of excellence and attention to detail.

For many women, taking up space hasn't been the norm. Those who dare to do so often face criticism, leading to silence and a world that misses out on their unique gifts. This shrinking might stem from personal trauma or from observing the women in your life growing up. But taking up space doesn't have to look the same for everyone. For some, it might mean using their voice to claim joy or pursuing a hobby. For others, it could mean making bold career moves or refusing to shrink in a room to make others comfortable.

A common challenge my patients face during healing is the discomfort their growth triggers in others, especially romantic partners who may not yet be on the same journey. This discomfort can tempt them to revert to old shrinking patterns. Here lies a pivotal choice: Return to the old story of shrinking or step into courage and continue choosing themselves.

Women possess unparalleled resilience and strength—if you've experienced or witnessed childbirth, you know this truth firsthand. The sheer capacity to endure, adapt, and persevere is a hallmark of feminine strength. Yet, this same strength often becomes a double-edged sword. Women are conditioned, consciously or not, to tolerate more than they should. We stay in situations that drain us, endure dynamics that stifle us, and carry burdens that are not ours to bear—all because we *can*. Our ability to tolerate discomfort, pain, and emotional weight is immense, and that very strength often keeps us stuck, believing we must endure rather than disrupt.

This resilience, while admirable, can create a cycle where we prioritize survival over thriving. We believe that to speak up, to ask for help, or to set boundaries is somehow selfish or weak. But true strength lies not in silent endurance but in recognizing when enough is enough. It is about channeling that resilience into advocating for ourselves, into saying, "I deserve better," and taking the steps to create change.

To harness this strength, we must reframe what it means to be strong. Strength doesn't mean carrying every burden alone. It means acknowledging when we are tired and finding the courage to say, "I need support." It means speaking up for our needs and breaking the silence that has too often muted our voices. By choosing to care for ourselves, we do not diminish our strength—we amplify it. This shift allows us to channel our tolerance into transformation, where we no longer merely survive but thrive, creating space for joy, healing, and the relationships we truly deserve.

Let us honor the strength that has brought us this far, not by continuing to tolerate, but by finding ways to use it to set boundaries, speak up, and care for ourselves unapologetically. True empowerment begins when we use our unparalleled capacity not just to endure, but to grow and create the life we deserve.

Choosing courage, though challenging, often inspires those around us to rise to meet our energy. It creates a ripple effect of healing that extends beyond the self. As you expand and take up space, you give others permission to do the same.

## The Framework for Healing

One way to begin the healing process is by incorporating simple, transformative daily habits, like those found in the 5M Model of daily transformation, to set the foundation for self-discovery and growth.

The 5M Model is a practical and approachable framework to support both your hormonal and emotional health. In the following chapters, we will explore each element of this model in depth, so you can seamlessly integrate these changes into your daily life. By focusing on the five pillars—Movement, Meals and Nutrition, Mindset, Morning/Evening Rituals, and the Mojo Mender—you can build a strong foundation for health habits that not only balance your hormones but also elevate your mood, boost your energy, and provide a reliable anchor when life feels overwhelming.

## The Pillars of the 5M Model

**Movement:** Moving your body in a way that aligns with your current season of life and the state of your nervous system is essential. If you're under constant stress and stuck in fight-or-flight mode, engaging in high-intensity workouts like marathon training or intense cardio might do more harm than good. These activities can further tax your adrenals and delay the results you're seeking. Instead, choose gentler forms of movement that soothe your body and activate your parasympathetic state—such as walking, yoga, or qigong. These practices not only reduce stress but also release endorphins, the feel-good hormones your body craves. Many women find that slowing down their workouts can actually help reduce hormonal belly weight, as their bodies finally feel safe enough to let go of stored fat.

**Meals:** Eating in a way that supports your hormones is key to giving your body the nutrients it needs to thrive. Hormonal health depends on balancing blood sugar levels, reducing inflammation, and nourishing your cells with the right macronutrients and micronutrients. Each meal becomes an opportunity to fuel your body for healing and growth. In later chapters, we'll dive into the kinds of foods that can help stabilize your hormones, including those rich in healthy fats, proteins, and fiber, while identifying foods to avoid that might disrupt your hormonal balance.

**Mindset:** Shifting into a positive mindset is a powerful tool for creating lasting change. By building self-awareness and resilience, you can better navigate life's challenges and reduce the stress that often drives hormonal imbalance. Mindset work involves adopting daily practices like journaling, gratitude exercises, or meditation to reframe limiting beliefs and focus on self-compassion and growth. A supportive mindset isn't just about silencing negative thoughts—it's about creating space for hope, motivation, and empowerment.

**Morning/Evening Rituals:** Establishing consistent rituals at the start and end of your day can have a profound impact on your health and well-being. Mornings set the tone for the day ahead, while evenings help your body wind down and prepare for rest. These rituals don't need to be complicated—simple practices like hydrating first thing in the morning, spending a few moments in gratitude, or unplugging from screens an hour before bed can signal to your body and mind that it's time to transition into a new phase of the day. These rituals also provide structure, which can help reduce stress and bring a sense of stability.

**Mojo Mender:** The practice of restoring connection, trust, and intimacy in your relationships as you heal your hormones and emotions. Just as your body responds to stress, nourishment, and movement, your relationships are deeply intertwined with your overall well-being. The way you show up in your closest connections—whether with a partner, family, or friendships—directly influences your hormonal health and emotional state.

When your nervous system is stuck in fight-or-flight mode, it becomes harder to communicate clearly, feel safe in intimacy, or receive love without resistance. Many women find that as they work on their movement, meals, mindset, and rituals, they begin to uncover unresolved emotional patterns that show up in their relationships—like difficulty setting boundaries, feeling unseen or unheard, or holding on to resentment. Mojo Mender is here to help bridge that gap, offering practical exercises to strengthen your connection to yourself and others, release old wounds, and create space for healthier, more fulfilling relationships.

Just like your body needs nourishment, your relationships need intentional care and healing to thrive. Throughout the healing plans, you'll find guided practices, reflective exercises, and tools to help you rebuild intimacy, trust, and communication—whether that's learning to speak your needs with confidence, releasing emotional baggage that keeps you stuck, or shifting the way you receive love and support.

By incorporating the 5M Model into your life, you'll create a sustainable and balanced approach to healing. Each component supports the others, weaving together a holistic system that empowers you to thrive, not just survive. This model will be your guide to rediscovering harmony in your hormones, emotions, and daily rhythms.

## Anchoring Your Treatment

When we choose to say no to one thing, we create space to say yes to something else. Setting boundaries—a skill unfamiliar to many of us—is an act of service to both our physical and emotional health. Often, we say yes out of obligation rather than joy, stretching ourselves thin and leaving little energy for what truly nourishes us. This is not to suggest rejecting everything or everyone; there are responsibilities we cannot avoid. But when our habits and choices begin to deplete our mind and body, it becomes vital to prioritize the decisions that restore and uplift us. For greater success with the following plans, having the capacity to choose yourself is going to be essential.

With any plan or commitment to change, give yourself at least three months to allow for lasting transformation and time for your body and mind to break the engrained cycles. This timeframe provides space for experimentation, self-reflection, and curiosity about what your body truly needs. Embracing this mindset of exploration helps you identify the choices that best support your well-being and lay the foundation for a healthier, more balanced life.

Before we dive into the specific plans tailored to each hormonal identity, I want to introduce you to the three foundational anchors of care I prioritize with every woman who sits in front of me. These anchors serve as the guiding principles for reconnecting with your body, emotions, and relationships and where these plans have been birthed from. First, take a moment to pause and reflect on two essential questions:

**What is the recurring theme of my discomfort?**

**What is my personal anchor?**

When finding the recurrent theme as yourself, what patterns, thoughts, habits, fights, or symptoms seem to replay in your life, whether monthly or during those overwhelming moments? Is there a recurring argument—perhaps with a loved one—that stems from unspoken resentment, bubbling to the surface when fluctuating hormones no longer let you suppress it? Is there an inner narrative you've been carrying, one that tears you down, that needs disrupting so you can start planting beliefs that build you up?

When finding your anchor, ask yourself: What feeling, emotion, or state do you need to be in to thrive? Is it peaceful, content, grounded, calm, or present? When you know that anchor, in your daily decisions with your health plan, you can ask yourself if the choices are taking you closer or further away from that anchor.

Understanding your hormonal identity and the recurring themes of discomfort in your life allows you to tailor your healing plan with intention and clarity. Knowing your anchor helps you stay consistent and committed to the plan. It's not just about addressing physical symptoms—it's about recognizing the cycles in your thoughts, emotions, and interactions that are deeply tied to your hormonal health and the state you are moving toward.

The first treatment anchor is **hormonal health**, which encompasses not only the physical aspects but also **mental and emotional well-being**. This includes modalities such as herbal remedies, targeted nutrition, movement, and repatterning the story, and, when appropriate, bioidentical hormone replacement therapy (BHRT).

Second is **detoxification**, a vital process that involves integrating daily habits to support the body's natural detox pathways, alongside more comprehensive detox programs conducted once or twice a year to clear deeper layers of toxins to make room for better communication between your hormones and your cells.

Third is **lifestyle and longevity**, where we establish sustainable daily habits and provide resources to empower you to take control of your health. These anchors form the foundation of a holistic and proactive approach to healing and thriving.

## Hormone Therapy

Bioidentical hormone replacement therapy (BHRT) can be a confusing topic, particularly in light of the Women's Health Initiative (WHI) study on synthetic hormone replacement therapy (HRT), which created widespread misunderstanding about hormone therapy. Since then, further research has clarified many of the nuances overlooked in that study, such as the type of hormone replacement used, and the specific criteria of the women included in the study population. Essentially, we now understand that relying solely on that single study to make health decisions is not enough.

To simplify the difference between BHRT and HRT, think of a key and a lock. BHRT is like a precisely crafted key that fits perfectly into the lock of your hormone receptors, turning smoothly and unlocking the balance your body needs. HRT, on the other hand, is like a similar-looking key that might slide into the lock but doesn't quite fit perfectly. It may jiggle or even partially turn, but it doesn't function as seamlessly, potentially leading to unintended effects. While this is a basic explanation of a more complex topic, the key idea is that BHRT, when guided by appropriate testing and symptom evaluation, can be a highly effective tool for improving a woman's physical and emotional health. Derived from natural sources like wild yam, BHRT is human-identical and can be administered in smaller, physiological doses (calibrated to match what the body needs at this stage of life) to achieve significant results.

In contrast, synthetic HRT, such as the hormones found in birth control, can cause drastic changes in how a woman feels. While some women experience benefits, others may endure negative side effects. Unfortunately, this area of medicine has not been studied as comprehensively as it deserves. I choose BHRT over HRT because its human-identical structure and low-dose application align more closely with the body's natural processes, often yielding remarkable outcomes. When combined with the holistic strategies we've discussed throughout this book, BHRT can be a true game changer for many women.

## Detox Essentials

Detoxification is essential for achieving optimal health. It starts with understanding how to open your emunctories—your body's natural elimination pathways—daily. This can be achieved through proper nutrition, herbs, supplements, and specific binders while also addressing the environmental toxins that disrupt your hormones and overall well-being. In today's world, detoxification isn't a luxury; it's a necessity. Both Ayurvedic and naturopathic medicine are rooted in the principle of detoxification, emphasizing the importance of helping the body release *ama*—toxins from the cells, body, brain, and mind. As discussed earlier, hormones struggle to communicate effectively when toxins and debris block their pathways. Similarly, the mind and emotions cannot find calm when the body feels congested and stuck.

Lifestyle and longevity habits offer a powerful way to take control of your health. These rituals don't need to be elaborate, and in the following plans, I will share simple practices you can incorporate into your daily life. However, if possible, investing in tools like an infrared sauna or cold-exposure setup can be transformative. These practices provide your body with opportunities to adapt to controlled stressors, a process known as *hormesis*. Just as your muscles grow stronger by adapting to the stress of exercise, exposing your body to alternating heat and cold helps build resilience and strengthens your stress response. The key, however, is to know when to push and when to rest. For someone in the midst of adrenal fatigue or burnout, adding more stress—even in a controlled way—can lead to greater imbalance, so timing and awareness are crucial.

Other tools, such as light therapy, specifically red and infrared light, offer both external and internal benefits. Externally, it can boost collagen production for healthier skin, while internally, it helps calm the nervous system, regulate your circadian rhythm, and promote deeper sleep and faster recovery from stress. Coffee enemas are another effective practice for detoxification, clearing the bowels of accumulated waste and promoting overall health.

Each habit carries its own unique benefits—whether it's detoxifying your body, strengthening your immune system, or balancing your hormones. Together, these habits give you the ability to cultivate greater vitality and resilience in your body.

At the end of the day, the simpler the plan, the greater the chance of success. The essence of all this is to help you reconnect with the foundational elements that humans need to thrive: love and connection. Eating nourishing foods, moving your body regularly, prioritizing quality sleep, and fostering meaningful social interactions and relationships are the key ingredients to a healthy and joyful life. Each of the modalities I've mentioned could fill a book on their own, and many experts have written extensively about them. My intention here is simply to plant these seeds so you can explore what resonates with you.

Remember, there is no one else like you—no one else carries the same stories, beliefs, or experiences that have shaped your journey to this moment. Embrace curiosity, ask questions, build your healing team, and confidently invite the universe to guide you on this path of self-discovery. You deserve it!

In the next three chapters, you will find a summary of different hormonal conditions and key considerations for addressing them, followed by specific plans tailored to your hormonal identity. You will gain access to simple tools you can use to heal your hormones, emotions, and relations. These plans are designed for you to begin incorporating them into your life right away. However, more specific elements—such as certain herbs, nutraceuticals, and bioidentical hormone replacement therapy (BHRT)—should be discussed with your healthcare provider to ensure they align with your unique needs and health goals.

CHAPTER 9

# Breaking the Cycle of Overdrive

## Plan A: Finding Calm for the Anxious Overachiever with the HER Method—When in Doubt, Start Here

This plan is designed for anyone who needs to reset their nervous system and find calm amid the chaos of daily life. It's also a great starting point if you're unsure where to begin. We've learned how pivotal stress is to the health of our hormones, emotions, and relationships, as well as its influence over our overall moodscape. By focusing on regulating the nervous system, you create space for all parts of yourself—mind, body, and soul—to start healing. This renewed energy allows you to peel back the deeper layers of past experiences and move confidently toward your future.

For this identity, where taming the mind often feels like an uphill battle, the treatment emphasizes retraining the nervous system as the foundation for hormonal balance. The goal is simple: Relax the body to quiet the mind, leading to days that feel both more energized and grounded. As your nervous system begins to activate its parasympathetic response and cortisol levels decrease, your sex hormones will have the chance to rebalance naturally. Commit to this approach for 90 days and witness the transformative shifts in your energy and overall well-being.

| 5M MODEL | TYPE | CONSIDERATIONS | THE WHY |
|---|---|---|---|
| Movement | Resistance training—lift heavy weights a few times a week<br>Yoga | Variation for this archetype is important to keep things exciting. She also needs something vigorous but not too taxing to get her out of her mind and into her body, in combination with softness to help regulate her nervous system. | To serve the nervous system, the goal here is to create more relaxation in the body while building strength. High intensity would further deplete the adrenal glands and keep the nervous system in a vigilant state, causing further depletion. |
| Meals and Nutrition | 3 whole-food meals a day with no snacking.<br>Supplements to support neurotransmitters like serotonin and GABA, and hormones like progesterone and cortisol regulation. Herbs to reset the nervous system. | She may tend to skip meals because of her busy schedule, so the priority is to create easy meals eaten at regular times to create stability in the nervous system. All supplemental and herbal support is geared toward replenishing the hormones. | The goal here is to create stability, routine, and trust in her ability to digest food and in her life—helping her to feel safe and in some level of control of her schedule and her health. |
| Mindset | Chanting—mantra or affirmation<br>Walking meditation<br>Humming | Incorporate a practice that can be done in the car, in the office, at pickup. Make it easy to establish a relationship with the mind. | Telling her to sit down for 30 minutes to meditate will create more anxiety. Giving her a tool that allows her to still and flow with her day empowers her. |
| Morning/ Evening Rituals | Habit stacking with positive self-awareness practices | Add a habit to the already existing routine, like when she is brushing her teeth. | This takes away any anxiety around adding something new to her day. As this becomes a part of her day, she will no longer think of it as separate but as something she always needed. |
| Mojo Mender | Exercises for more calm | Giving herself time to connect creates safety and trust. | This allows her to be softer with herself and others. |

## Movement as Medicine

For the Anxious Overachiever, tension isn't just a mental or emotional experience—it's something her body holds on to, often in ways she doesn't realize. The drive to constantly perform, stay ahead, and meet expectations—whether at work, in relationships, or even in her personal health journey—creates an ongoing state of physical contraction. This identity thrives on structure, control, and achieving results, but this very tendency to "hold it all together" can translate into unconscious muscle tension, particularly in the pelvic floor.

The pelvic floor is a direct reflection of the nervous system's ability to shift between **fight-or-flight (sympathetic mode) and rest-and-digest (parasympathetic mode)**. When stress hormones like cortisol dominate, the pelvic floor muscles tighten as a protective mechanism—whether from past trauma, ongoing stress, or the mental weight of trying to do it all. Over time, this chronic holding pattern can create:

- **Hormonal imbalances** (due to poor circulation and communication between the brain and reproductive organs)
- **Pelvic pain or discomfort** (even without an underlying medical issue)
- **Irregular or painful periods** (caused by restricted blood flow and stagnation)
- **Sexual dysfunction or low libido** (because tension in the pelvic floor can create numbness or hypersensitivity)
- **Digestive issues like constipation or bloating** (due to pressure on the intestines and improper engagement of core muscles)

The science behind this connection is profound. The **pelvic floor is deeply linked to the brain's stress and emotion centers**, specifically:

- The **periaqueductal gray (PAG) area** in the midbrain plays a role in regulating pelvic floor muscles and modulating fear and anxiety. It is influenced by the **amygdala** (the brain's fear center) and the **hypothalamus** (the master regulator of hormones).
- When the amygdala senses stress, it signals the **hypothalamus** to release stress hormones, reinforcing tension in the body—especially in the pelvic floor, which is innervated by the sacral parasympathetic motor neurons.
- Over time, this creates a cycle where unresolved stress and emotional repression lead to hormonal imbalances, menstrual irregularities, and even fertility challenges.

## MORNING YOGA ROUTINE

Here I have chosen postures that are easy and create calm in your nervous system. You don't need an hour to feel grounded in your body, just a little movement can go a long way. Create your sacred space and give yourself a moment to connect with your body.

You can end the practice by lying on your belly with your cheek to the floor, letting your breath regulate and body relax. I always end my practice with a meditation or some breathwork to help set up my day from a place of calm. Remember, this can literally be like a minute! Here is an affirmation that you could also use: "I choose to walk my day with ease."

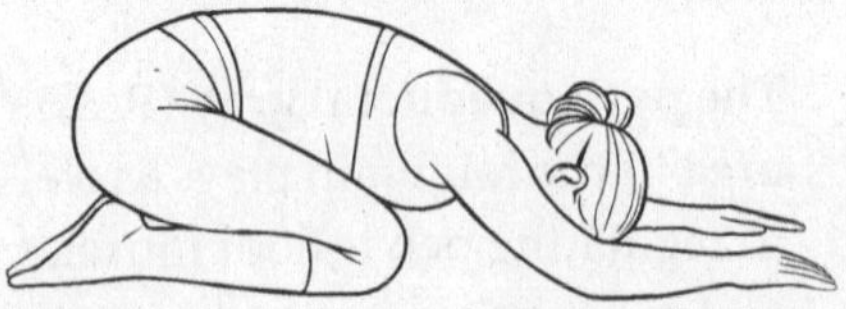

### Child's Pose (Balasana)

Start your practice in child's pose with your knees apart, your forehead on the ground, and arms stretched overhead. Take a deep breath in through your nose to the count of 4, hold, and then let out an exhale through your mouth with a deep sigh to the count of 8. Repeat 3 times. While in this posture, create an intention for your practice.

### Cat Cow Pose (Marjaryasana and Bitilasana)

Come onto your hands and knees with knees hip width apart and your hands shoulder width apart. Inhale and lift your chin up, flexing the spine down into Cow and then exhale, bringing the chin back toward your chest and rounding your back into Cat. Feel the spaces between your vertebrae opening as you move through these postures. Continue for 1 to 3 minutes.

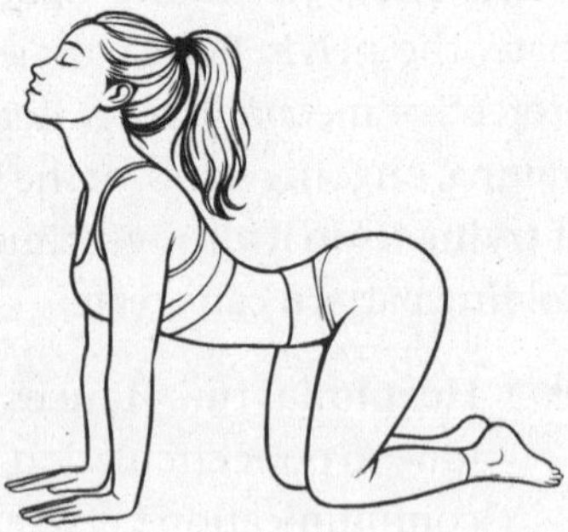

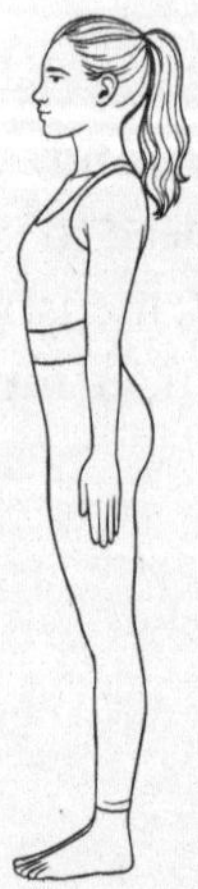

### Mountain Pose (Tadasana)

Come standing with your feet rooted to the ground and hip distance apart. Lift the inner arches of your feet up and root down on all four corners of your feet. Draw your inner thighs back, lengthen your torso, broaden the upper back, and draw your belly in and up. Draw your shoulder blades down your back and broaden your collar bones. Arms straight and palms facing forward, and have your chin parallel to the floor. Soften your gaze and breathe long and deep.

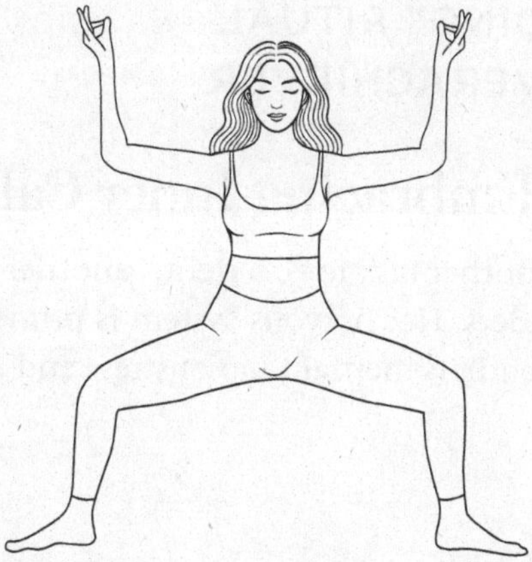

## Goddess Pose with Prayer (Utkata Konasana)

Come into goddess pose with your feet pointing out, shoulders relaxed, and arms wide and open. On the inhale, open your arms, and on the exhale, bring your hands into prayer with palms together in front of your heart center.

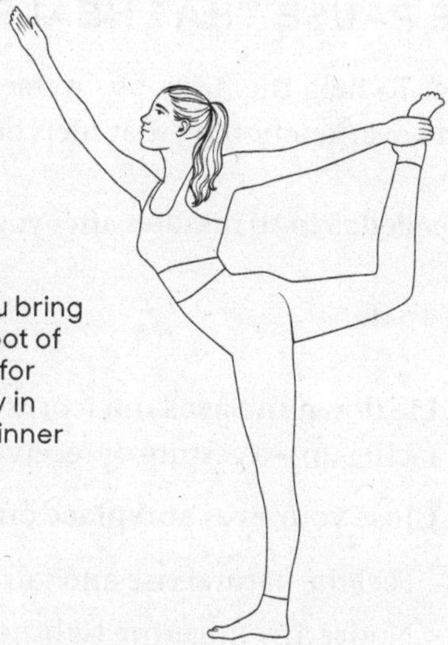

## Dancer's Pose (Natarajasana)

Steady yourself on one foot. Lift the other leg as you bring the same hand back to grab the inner part of the foot of the lifted leg. Bring the opposite arm in front of you for balance. Relax your shoulders and create neutrality in your hips. Don't forget to breathe and tap into your inner dancer! Repeat on the opposite side.

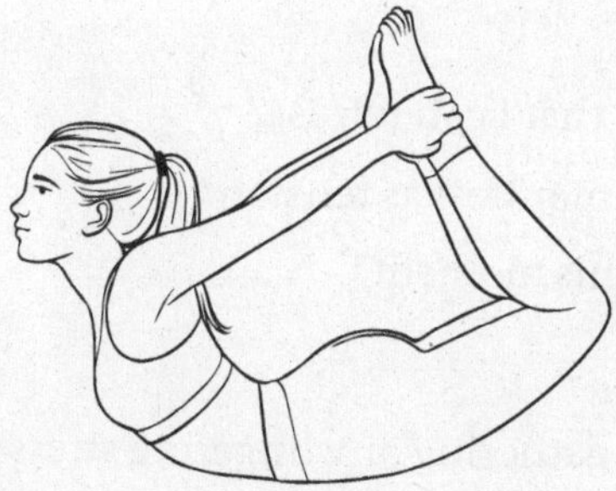

## Bow Pose (Dhanurasana)

Come lying on your belly and place your forehead to the ground with your arms by your side. Take a few deep breaths and begin to bend your knees and lift your lower legs toward your sit bones, grabbing each ankle with your hands and pulling your chest up and open. Keep your chin tucked in. On the inhale, lift up and on the exhale relax. Repeat for 1 to 3 minutes.

## POST-YOGA "UNWINDING" RITUAL FOR THE ANXIOUS OVERACHIEVER

# Releasing the Mental Load & Embracing Inner Calm

For the Anxious Overachiever, yoga may feel like another task to "do right," another place where she unconsciously pushes instead of surrenders. Her nervous system is primed for action, but healing requires her to step out of the endless mental loop of stress and into a state of presence.

## EXERCISE: "THE PAUSE THAT HEALS"—RELEASING THE MENTAL GRIP

**Purpose:** To help the Anxious Overachiever break free from the overthinking, overplanning, and overfunctioning that fuels her stress and retrain her nervous system to rest.

**Time needed:** 5 to 10 minutes after yoga

**How to do it:**

1. **Lie down in Savasana** (corpse pose) with your arms by your sides, palms facing up—a gesture of receiving rather than controlling.
2. **Close your eyes and place one hand on your heart and one on your belly.**
   - Feel the natural rise and fall of your breath.
   - Notice any lingering tightness in your jaw, shoulders, or belly, and allow it to soften.
3. **Silently ask:**
   - What is one thought I am gripping on to that I can release?
   - Where in my body do I feel this thought manifest as tension?
   - What would it feel like to let go, just for this moment?
4. **Release the breath.**
   - Inhale through your nose for **4 seconds**, gathering any lingering stress in your body.

- Hold for **4 seconds**, feeling where tension lingers.
- Exhale audibly through your mouth for **6 seconds**, imagining the stress dissolving like mist.
- Repeat for **5 rounds**, each time surrendering a little more.

5. **Close with an affirmation.**

- Whisper or say aloud:

  *I do not have to prove my worth. I am enough just as I am.*

  *I allow myself to rest without guilt.*

  *I am safe in the stillness.*

---

## INTEGRATION: THE "ONE-MINUTE RESET" PRACTICE

Throughout the day, when you catch yourself spiraling into stress, overscheduling, or feeling overwhelmed, you can use a one-minute reset:

- **Pause.**
- **Take one deep breath.**
- **Release one thing—an unnecessary thought, task, or expectation.**

This microinterruption helps retrain your brain to detach from urgency and step into ease.

**Why it works:**

- Regulates the nervous system by shifting from a high-cortisol state to a rest-and-repair mode.
- Breaks the stress cycle by rewiring the belief that you must always be doing to be worthy.
- Creates a pause for emotional processing rather than immediate action.

This ritual trains your mind and body to embrace calm without guilt, creating space for healing, connection, and presence.

## Meals and More

How you feed your body is deeply connected to how you nurture your emotions and hormones. We now know that the tiny organisms in your gut—the microbiome—play a significant role in your mental, emotional, and physical health. Understanding this gut-brain connection is essential, but even more critical is learning how to nourish this connection with foods your body can properly digest. Remember, how you digest your food reflects how you digest your life.

When you're overwhelmed or anxious, your body shifts its focus to survival, effectively shutting down digestion. Staying in this state for an extended period often leads to chronic gut challenges like constipation, diarrhea, bloating, and more. These physical discomforts then create a vicious cycle that impacts your mind, body, and hormones.

For those stuck in a cycle of anxious stress, I often turn to the principles of Ayurvedic medicine, specifically the concept of *prakriti*—your innate constitution, or doshas. The doshas describe unique tendencies, traits, and susceptibilities that provide insight into how and what you should eat. For example, we focus here on the *vata* dosha, which governs movement in the body and mind. When vata becomes imbalanced, it can lead to chaotic, frantic energy and digestive disruptions. Pacifying vata through proper nutrition can help restore balance and calm to both body and mind.

To dive deeper into this concept, I highly recommend reading *Prakriti: Your Ayurvedic Constitution* by Dr. Robert E. Svoboda. Meanwhile, I'll share key nutritional principles from the book to guide you in selecting foods that support your body when you're feeling overwhelmed and anxious.

## General Rules

1. Eat a variety of seasonal whole foods.
2. Eat organic fruits and vegetables, especially those on the Dirty Dozen list, created by the Environmental Working Group, of produce items most contaminated with pesticides.
3. Avoid genetically modified ingredients.
4. Pause to eat your meals without distractions, especially screens.
5. Give thanks to the food. This practice alone can change the charge around the food and your ability to digest it.

General rules include eating a variety of whole foods, no sugar, and limited dairy and gluten. The most important thing to remember is sourcing organic food, since the pesticides on fruits and vegetables mimic estrogen and act as hormone disruptors. What disrupts the digestion will disrupt the hormones and disrupt the emotions. Quick and easy 30-minute meals that focus on grounding foods for your nervous system help you feel calm. Because the Anxious Overachiever identity has more digestive upset, the focus is on foods that are easy to digest and warming in nature. Feeding your microbiome meals filled with nourishment will help reduce any inflammation in the digestive system, allowing neurotransmitters like serotonin to provide the calm your nervous system needs.

| FOODS TO AVOID | FOODS TO INCLUDE |
|---|---|
| **Grains:** Any that are drying, but can have on occasion if you add ghee and other healthy fats to them<br>Buckwheat<br>Corn<br>Millet<br>Rye | **Grains:** Make sure to have variation, and best eaten at lunch<br>Organic rice<br>Organic oats<br>Organic wheat (if tolerated) |
| **Vegetables:** Raw<br>Especially tomatoes<br>Spinach<br>Eggplant<br>Peppers | **Vegetables:** Cooked<br>All vegetables, especially cooked. Below are some of the best:<br>Asparagus<br>Beets<br>Carrots<br>Celery<br>Garlic<br>Green beans<br>Okra<br>Onion<br>Parsnips<br>Radishes<br>Rutabagas<br>Turnips<br>Sweet potatoes |
| **Fruit:** Avoid any that are drying and astringent<br>Cranberry<br>Apples<br>Pomegranate<br>All dried fruit<br>Unripe banana | **Fruit:** To be consumed in the summer and minimal in other seasons<br>Apricots<br>Avocado<br>Banana<br>Berries<br>Cherries<br>Coconut<br>Soaked dates and figs<br>Grapefruit<br>Grapes<br>Lemons<br>Mangoes<br>Melons<br>Nectarines<br>Oranges<br>Papaya<br>Peaches<br>Pears<br>Pineapple<br>Plums |

| | |
|---|---|
| **Fish/Meats/Dairy:** Can be grounding for this state if you are not a vegetarian/vegan. Avoid overindulgence, and always make sure it is organic to avoid hormone disruption.<br>Take care with shellfish<br>Fried eggs | **Fish/Meats/Dairy:** Can consume all if digestion and ethics allow. |
| **Legumes:** Avoid overindulgence due to nitrogenous waste products in the body, like other protein sources.<br>Peanuts<br>Tofu | **Legumes:** Should be cooked with turmeric, cumin, coriander, ginger, garlic, healthy oil. Should also be soaked overnight.<br>Mung beans (best)<br>Split peas/beans (easier to digest)<br>Black lentils<br>Red lentils<br>Chickpeas<br>Organic non-GMO tofu in moderation |
| **Nuts and Seeds/Oils:**<br>Raw almonds with skin<br>Excess sesame seeds<br>Safflower oil | **Nuts and Seeds/Oils:**<br>Soaked almonds<br>Pumpkin seeds<br>Most nuts and seeds (unless mentioned under "Foods to Avoid")<br>Sesame oil<br>Almond oil |

SAMPLE MENU

# Breakfast Options

## Warming Hormone-Supporting Drink

1 cup whole A2 grass-fed and organic milk or alternative milk of your choice, warmed up (A2 milk contains a form of the protein beta-casein that is easier to digest)
2 soaked dates
1 tablespoon ground flaxseed
1 tablespoon hemp seeds
1 tablespoon ashwagandha powder (optional)
1 tablespoon peeled almonds
½ teaspoon cacao powder
Cinnamon and allspice, to taste

Blend the ingredients together. Add cinnamon and allspice to taste.

## Warm Oatmeal Delight Breakfast

1 to 2 tablespoons ghee, divided
1 cup gluten-free organic steel-cut oats
½ teaspoon cinnamon
1 pinch cumin
½ teaspoon cardamom powder
A few cloves
1 pinch nutmeg
2 cups filtered water
1 teaspoon hemp seeds
1 teaspoon ground flaxseed
1 teaspoon ashwagandha powder (optional)
½ teaspoon shredded ginger
1 to 2 teaspoons nut butter of choice
Maple syrup or honey for sweetening (optional)

Add 1 tablespoon of ghee to a pot over medium-low heat. Add the oats and all the spices except ginger. In a separate bowl, mix the ashwaghanda (if using) with 1 tablespoon of ghee and add to the pot with 2 cups of water. Simmer for about 10 minutes or until the oatmeal has the consistency you like. Then top with ginger, seeds, and nut butter. You can add maple syrup, honey, or a sweetener of your choice here, as desired.

# Lunch

## Mung Bean Noodle Stir-Fry with Almond Butter Sauce

One 200-gram (approximately 7-ounce) box mung bean noodles (like Explore Cuisine—they have one with mung bean and edamame)
2 tablespoon avocado oil
1 leek, chopped
2 to 3 cloves garlic, chopped
1 tablespoon minced fresh ginger root
½ to 1 teaspoon sea salt
1 head broccoli, chopped
2 carrots, shredded
1 sweet red pepper, thinly sliced
½ cup shredded red cabbage
1 bunch parsley

**For the sauce:**

½ cup almond butter
¼ cup filtered water
3 tablespoons rice vinegar
2 tablespoons toasted sesame oil
1 to 2 cloves garlic
1 teaspoon minced fresh ginger root
4 tablespoons tamari
1 tablespoon maple syrup (optional—I don't find the need for it, usually)

Boil the noodles as instructed on the box.

Add 2 tablespoons of avocado oil and the leeks, garlic, ginger, and salt to a pan. Cook for a minute over medium heat, then add the broccoli and cook slightly. Then add in the rest of the veggies except the parsley. The idea is to warm them slightly but not overcook them. Once cooked to where you desire, add in the cooked noodles and sauce. For the sauce, add all the ingredients to a blender and blend until you get the consistency you like. You may need a little extra water. Toss together and top with the parsley.

# Dinner

## Lentil Coconut Curry

1 tablespoon ghee, plus more for serving
1 teaspoon cumin seeds
1 white onion, chopped
A few slices ginger root, chopped
4 cloves garlic, chopped
1 tomato, chopped
1 teaspoon salt
1 teaspoon garam masala
1 teaspoon cumin powder
1 teaspoon paprika
¾ teaspoon turmeric
1 cup red lentils, soaked overnight
One 13.5-ounce (400 ml) can coconut milk
4 cups filtered water
1 bunch cilantro, chopped
1 bunch spinach, chopped

Put 1 tablespoon ghee and cumin seeds in a pot on medium heat. Cook for a minute and add the onions and ginger. Once the onions are translucent, add in the garlic, tomato, and salt. Cook for 1 minute and add the rest of the spices. Cook for a few minutes and add the lentils, coconut milk, and water. Let simmer on medium-low heat for 20 to 25 minutes. If you find the mixture is getting too thick, you can add more water. Once the curry is done, add the cilantro and spinach, and taste to see if it needs more salt. When eating the curry, pour a generous amount of ghee in your bowl.

## Herbs

Choosing the right herbs to support your parasympathetic nervous system can be a game changer when it comes to easing the overwhelm that comes from being stuck in a constant state of fight or flight. Stress has a profound impact on your body, hijacking your ability to rest, restore, and regulate your hormones. Incorporating herbs specifically targeted to calm your nervous system can help bring your body back into balance, alleviating feelings of anxiety, exhaustion, and burnout. These herbs not only help regulate stress responses but also nourish and support your hormones, allowing your body to function more optimally.

When selecting herbs, it's important to consult with a functional physician or herbalist to determine the best choices and dosing tailored to your unique needs. This ensures that you're using them effectively and safely while reaping their full benefits. Adaptogenic herbs like ashwagandha can help your body better adapt to stress, while nervine herbs like lemon balm calm your mind and promote a sense of relaxation. These herbs work synergistically to soothe frazzled nerves and provide nourishment for your adrenal glands, which are often overworked in high-stress states.

Incorporating these herbs into your daily routine can be as simple as sipping on herbal teas, adding tinctures to your water, or integrating capsules into your supplement plan. Over time, they help you cultivate resilience, calm your nervous system, and restore balance to your hormones—all while supporting your emotional and physical well-being.

| NAME OF HERB | ACTION |
|---|---|
| Chaste tree (*Vitex agnus-castus* berry) | Increases secretion of luteinizing hormone and favors progesterone, relieving your anxiety. |
| Licorice root | Hormone balancing and adrenal supporting. Not to be used with hypertension or if you are dealing with water retention and swelling. Can act to increase or decrease estrogenic effects depending on what your body needs. Giving you more energy and vitality to help downregulate the overwhelm. |
| Ashwagandha | Ayurvedic herb acts as an adaptogen and supports the HPA axis to reduce stress reactions in the body and mind. Also shown to reduce depletion of cortisol under times of stress. Helps with nervous exhaustion and is nurturing for the mind while supporting sleep. |
| Skullcap | A nervine with the capacity to calm the nerves and promote relaxation in the body and mind. |
| *Schisandra chinensis* | A warm tonic and adaptogenic herb and is high in vitamins C and E. In Chinese medicine, it is thought to "quiet the spirit and calm the heart." |
| Lemon balm (*Melissa officinalis*) | Calming for your nervous system and reduces impact of anxiety on your physical body. |
| *Ziziphus jujuba* | Reduces anxiety and promotes sleep. |

## Vitamins and Minerals

For the Anxious Overachiever, daily habits can often unknowingly drain the body of the essential vitamins and minerals needed for hormonal balance and emotional regulation. High stress levels, frequent consumption of caffeine or alcohol, and constant exposure to environmental toxins compound the depletion of these crucial nutrients. The demands of a busy life can push you into overdrive, leading to a state where your body is forced to borrow from its reserves just to keep you functioning, leaving little left for repair and restoration.

Stress, in particular, places a significant burden on the adrenal glands, increasing the need for key nutrients like magnesium, B vitamins, and zinc—all of which are vital for producing stress hormones, stabilizing your mood, and supporting energy levels. Alcohol and caffeine, often relied upon as coping mechanisms, further rob the body of these nutrients, making the cycle of depletion even more pronounced. Environmental toxins, from polluted air to processed foods, create oxidative stress in the body, demanding higher levels of antioxidants and minerals to combat their effects.

The result? A constant state of "running on empty" that leaves you feeling fatigued, anxious, and more susceptible to burnout. Understanding how your choices impact your body's reserves is the first step to breaking this cycle. By incorporating replenishing habits—nutrient-dense meals, targeted supplementation, hydration, and mindful movement—you can begin to restore what's been lost. These small but impactful changes will not only support your hormones and neurotransmitters but also improve your ability to manage stress, regulate emotions, and ultimately sustain the high performance you strive for without depleting yourself in the process.

| NAME | ACTIONS |
|---|---|
| Magnesium taurate, glycinate, threonate, and malate | These types of magnesium help support in relaxing the nervous system and aid in more restful sleep. They can help reduce the impact of stress and anxiety. |
| Zinc and Copper | Zinc is crucial for balanced female reproduction and healthy hormone production of progesterone, while copper is connected to estrogen. You don't need very much copper—just a slight amount—and you want to be mindful of too much if you have a copper IUD. |
| Vitamins $B_5$ and $B_6$ | $B_5$ is needed for adrenal health and balance, while $B_6$ is necessary for the synthesis of many neurotransmitters to support healthy moods. |
| Gamma-linolenic acid | Lowers inflammation and helps in the production of your hormones and gives a youthful glow to your skin, which is a total bonus! |
| Gamma-aminobutyric acid (GABA) | I find this especially helpful in the last half of the cycle. It acts as an inhibitory neurotransmitter to help calm your brain, emotions, and body. |

| | |
|---|---|
| Amino acids | These are the backbone of your cells and hormones and needed for any process to occur efficiently. |
| Chromium | Taken with meals to help regulate insulin function and blood sugar control to reduce the weight gain that comes from the excess cortisol and stress. |
| 5-hydroxytryptophan (5-HTP) | Precursor to serotonin. The neurotransmitter that helps you feel calm and connected, lowers anxiety, and even relaxes the digestive system. |
| Probiotics with strains *Lactobacillus rhamnosus* and *Bifidobacterium longum* | *Lactobacillus* helps activate GABA, a calming neurotransmitter, and *Bifidobacterium* has anxiolytic effects and supports the gut-brain connection. |

## Mindset Reset

Once you recognize the patterns your mind holds, you can access practices to help shift that state, freeing yourself from the grip of the monkey mind and its games. This reset strengthens the communication system between your brain and hormones. For the Anxious Overachiever, the busy mind often reinforces fears and worries, which can eventually escalate into anger. This default state serves as both a protective mechanism and a coping strategy for the mental overwhelm she carries. A helpful mantra to guide her through this habitual state is: *I choose to use this anger to fuel action and step into acceptance.*

The mind often clings to familiarity, resisting change to feel safe, which can trigger emotions like anger when life feels disrupted. For someone who feels locked and stuck in her thoughts and emotions, moving meditation becomes a powerful tool for transformation. Here, movement serves as both meditation and medicine, creating the shift needed to break free from these mental loops.

Commit yourself to doing a **"worry walk"** every day. This can be the few minutes you have walking from the car to your destination or as you walk your kids to school, or some time walking in nature. Here you get to talk to your mind about all the worries of the day, list them all out, and after every statement of worry, transform it into a win. Here's an example, "I'm worried I am not doing enough for the kids"—the win, "How lucky are they to have a mother that questions if she is doing enough for them, wow, I have the capacity to give them so much love!" Speak to your worry, speak to your anger, speak to your soul.

Becoming aware that the worry in your mind is temporary is a powerful step. That worry cannot be changed without taking different action—and this action doesn't need to be grand. It can be as simple as humming your favorite tune or chanting the mantra *Shanti, shanti, shanti* (peace, peace, peace). This seemingly small act activates and tones your vagus nerve, the longest nerve in your body, often called the "wanderer" because it extends throughout your body, impacting multiple organs. As we discussed in Chapter 7, by improving vagal tone, you enhance the expression of your parasympathetic nervous system—your body's rest, digest, and healing system. This shift reduces the impact of stress on your body, supporting the regulation of your hormones and emotions.

To help protect your nervous system and start your day with calm, you can use the **Meditation of Golden Light**. This practice creates a foundation for resilience and peace throughout your day.

*Sit in a comfortable seat or come lying down with your knees bent and low back rooted to the floor. Place your hands on your heart center. Close your eyes and take a deep breath in through your nose, expanding your belly and feeling the expansion of your heart beneath the palms of your hands. Exhale and allow the belly to go back to your spine. Continue with this breath. With each inhale imagine a golden light warming your hands as it shines out from your heart. On each exhale imagine that light expanding and becoming larger and larger with each breath until you can feel it covering your entire body. Notice the warmth and protection it provides as it encloses your body with light, warmth, strength, love, and protection. Once you feel that light expanded all over your being, rub your hands together and bring them to your eyes. Cup your eyes with your hands and say to yourself,* ***"It is in this present moment I heal, it is in this present moment I am free."*** *Then slowly open your eyes and lower your hands to your heart.*

## Morning and Evening Bliss

The moments just after waking from the dream world and the moments right before drifting into it at night set the tone for your entire day and the quality of your sleep. These moments influence how you feel emotionally, your energy and motivation levels, the balance of your hormones, and how steady you feel in your body. Rituals are essential in cultivating trust in yourself and your body. They act as anchors, especially during times of chaos when it feels like everything is falling apart. Having these intentional moments helps you feel centered, grounded, and secure, offering a sense of safety and peace.

Below is a list of rituals designed to support your nervous system, helping you feel calm and grounded in the morning and restful and ready for sleep at night. Start by choosing one ritual from each list, and as these practices become part of your daily routine, you can begin to layer in more. A helpful tip is to stack a new ritual with an existing habit—for example, humming while in the shower.

# Morning

### While still in bed:

1. Right when you wake up, say a word of gratitude.
2. Bring your knees into your chest and do a few seconds of Breath of Fire, a rhythmic, rapid breathing technique through the nose—passive inhales and active exhales are equal in length, powered by a quick pumping of the navel just below the belly button. This helps to wake up your digestion so you can have a bowel movement right in the morning.

### After you are up:

1. Drink warm water with a pinch of salt.
2. After brushing your teeth, gargle and swish around your mouth some sesame oil for as long as you can. About 15 to 20 minutes, or start with just a few. You can do this while you are getting your morning ready. This strengthens the gums and teeth while also increasing your vagal tone.
3. Give yourself a self-massage with sesame oil while stating an affirmation you need to help you feel steady. Below is a list of affirmations you can choose from, or you can get creative and create your own!

### Your morning affirmation . . .

1. I am not my thoughts and emotions; I am my choices.
2. I am enough.
3. I can be powerful and soft.
4. I can choose ease.
5. I am flaw-some!

# Evening

**Before going to bed:**

1. Carve out time to be off screens and do something you love: a puzzle, knitting, writing, reading, listening to music.
2. What gives you joy, and how can you use a few minutes before bed to nourish your soul? I get it, in the moment it might feel like watching a show and sitting on the couch is all you can do. So, if that is what you need, sister, you go for it, and all I ask is that you wear some blue-light blockers to begin the process of telling your brain sleep is coming.

**While in bed:**

1. Make a statement of gratitude for yourself. What did you do today that you are proud of? Just one! I know you can find it in yourself to see your brilliance!
2. Apply some sesame oil on your hands and feet and the below *marma* points to help your nervous system reset and relax. Marma points are pockets of energy, like acupuncture points that help regulate your nervous system.

   Marma point 1: *Adhipati*—located at your crown, essentially the center of your head. Apply a few drops of sesame oil there and massage in a circular motion.

   Marma point 2: *Talahridaya*—located in the middle of the soles of your feet. Apply a few drops of sesame oil and massage in a circular motion.

## From Overdoing to Overflowing—Relationship Edition

The Anxious Overachiever carries a deep sense of urgency, a feeling that if she doesn't do everything—immediately—things will fall apart. This intensity bleeds into her relationships, often making them feel strained, distant, or overly demanding. While she may deeply love her partner, friends, or family, her exhaustion and stress make true connection difficult. The journey to healing is not just about supporting her hormones; it is also about learning how to let love and support in while breaking the cycle of overdoing.

When the nervous system is in overdrive, it interprets love, rest, and intimacy as secondary to survival. For her, relaxation is foreign, asking for help is uncomfortable, and vulnerability feels like a risk. But relationships thrive when there is room for softness, trust, and connection. This section offers strategies to bridge the gap between her stress and her relationships—giving her tools to reconnect while healing.

## The Power of the Pause: Releasing Reactivity in Relationships

When under stress, the Anxious Overachiever can be short-tempered, critical, and impatient—not out of malice, but because her nervous system is overloaded. If she has a history of feeling unheard or needing to prove herself, she may become defensive or emotionally withdrawn when her partner doesn't immediately respond in the way she expects.

The **"Pause and Breathe" Method**: When emotions start to escalate, pause before responding. Take three slow, deep breaths and ask:

- Am I responding from stress or from my truth?
- What do I actually need in this moment?
- Can I communicate that with kindness instead of urgency?

This gives the nervous system a moment to shift out of fight or flight, allowing the Anxious Overachiever to respond rather than react in her relationships.

## LEARNING TO RECEIVE: THE INTIMACY RESET EXERCISE

The Anxious Overachiever is often the giver in relationships—she anticipates needs before they are spoken, takes on more than her fair share, and rarely allows herself to receive—often out of the need to control. This imbalance can create resentment, exhaustion, and distance in her relationships.

**Couple's exercise:**

- Set aside 15 minutes in the evening where a woman practices receiving only.
- Her partner asks: "How can I support you right now?"
- She must choose one small thing—this could be a hug, words of affirmation, or even a simple, "I just need you to sit with me."
- The key is learning to accept support without guilt, justification, or reciprocation.

This small act of receiving resets her nervous system, teaching her body that she is not alone in the weight she carries.

## TOUCH AS MEDICINE: THE 30-SECOND CONNECTION RITUAL

When stress is high, intimacy often takes a backseat. The Anxious Overachiever may feel disconnected from her body, making physical connection feel like another task rather than something enjoyable.

**Try this 30-second practice to reset connection daily:**

- Before bed or in the morning, spend 30 seconds holding hands with your partner, hugging, or placing a hand on each other's heart.
- Breathe together—slow, deep inhales and exhales.
- No talking—just presence.

Physical connection calms the nervous system, lowers cortisol, and increases oxytocin (the bonding hormone). This simple act can rebuild trust, safety, and connection without requiring long conversations or effort.

## REFLECTION EXERCISE:

- Ask: How do I feel when I am not being "productive" in my relationship?
- Ask: Do I feel guilty resting? Unworthy when I'm not doing enough?
- Write down 3 ways you can receive love without effort. For example:
    - Letting your partner make decisions for a day.
    - Letting go of the need to control the schedule for a weekend.
    - Allowing someone to care for you without feeling like you owe them something in return.

This practice reteaches your nervous system that love is safe, effortless, and not something that needs to be constantly "achieved."

**Saying No Without Guilt: Boundary Practice**

Boundaries are an essential part of healing for the Anxious Overachiever. Because she feels responsible for everything, she often says yes when she means no, takes on too much, or feels resentful when people don't recognize how much she's doing.

## THE SOFT NO EXERCISE

- If saying no feels impossible, try:
    - "I'd love to, but I don't have the capacity right now."
    - "I can't commit to that, but I appreciate you thinking of me."
- Recognize that setting a boundary is not rejection—it is self-preservation.
- The more you strengthen this muscle, the more energy you will have for the things that actually nourish you.

## The Overachiever's Love Language: Shifting from "Doing" to "Being"

An Anxious Overachiever often expresses love by doing—acts of service, planning, taking on responsibilities. But relationships need balance. If she always feels like she has to earn love through effort, she may miss out on the simple joy of being loved as she is.

Healing hormones isn't just about food and supplements—it's about shifting patterns, including those in relationships. When the Anxious Overachiever learns to calm her stress response, receive love, communicate without urgency, and set boundaries without guilt, she begins to experience relationships as a source of support, not stress.

These practices are not about adding more to her plate—they are about taking things off, making space, and allowing her to heal in a way that feels safe, supported, and sustainable.

Because love isn't something to be earned through exhaustion—it's something to be felt, received, and trusted.

CHAPTER 10

# Breaking the Cycle of Pleasing

## Plan B: Empowering the Silent Struggler with the HER Method

This plan is for rebuilding and remembering—to remind the Silent Struggler of the immense strength she possesses and the joy she is inherently deserving of. The Silent Struggler often depletes her vitality in the pursuit of pleasing others, leaving her feeling drained and disconnected. There is a fragility in her body and mind that requires nurturing, rebuilding, and strengthening. This is the plan for when getting out of bed feels like an impossible task, when her immune system reacts to every little trigger—whether it's a certain food or a minor environmental change—when circulation is poor, and when hormonal deficiencies leave her feeling imbalanced and low.

For the woman who silently struggles, this plan addresses her unspoken battles—the exhaustion, the guilt of feeling weak, the fear of asking for help, and the overwhelming desire to just feel like herself again. These silent struggles often stem from a deep-rooted pattern of neglecting her own needs while prioritizing everyone else's. This plan begins by creating a safe space to prioritize herself, even if it feels unfamiliar and uncomfortable at first. It emphasizes nourishing her body with the right nutrients, stabilizing her energy, and giving her the tools to set boundaries that foster healing.

Physically, she may experience thyroid dysfunction, chronic anemia, and a persistent sense of disconnect and low motivation. These symptoms are clues that her body is crying out for care. The focus here is on rebuilding her vitality step by step—nourishing her hormones, supporting her immune system, and creating more resilience through small, sustainable changes. Strengthening her sense of self and reminding her of the power she has always carried will also help her establish healthy boundaries, both physically and emotionally.

This is not just about addressing the physical symptoms; it is also about reconnecting her with her inner strength and her ability to find joy. By supporting her nervous system, boosting her circulation, and gently addressing hormonal imbalances, she will find the resilience to reclaim her health and rediscover her identity—one that is no longer tied to self-sacrifice but to empowerment and self-love.

| 5M MODEL | TYPE | CONSIDERATIONS | THE WHY |
|---|---|---|---|
| Movement | Yoga and qigong | This identity or stage requires a soft approach to rebuild strength and trust back in her body. Yoga postures help bring awareness and resilience back into the body. | Because she is in a state of depletion, anything too vigorous can create further stress and depletion in the body. However, we still want to choose postures that remind her of her strength. |
| Meals and Nutrition | Whole foods that will stimulate her mind and awaken her digestion: 2 to 3 meals a day with no snacks in between | There is a sluggishness in this identity, so heavy foods are to be avoided. We want dense nutrients. | This identity is so used to feeding others first that she often is eating scraps from the kid's plates. So, it will take practice and patience to reprogram her relationship to nourishment. |
| Mindset | Meditation<br>Creativity<br>Chanting<br>Singing | Use her voice to chant or sing to practice projecting her voice. Doing something creative that she loves will ignite passion and energy inside of her. | This identity often has difficulty using her voice and voicing her opinion or boundaries. Creating a practice to do so will help retrain the trust in your intuition and voice once again. |
| Morning/Evening Rituals | Setting aside time, even just a few minutes in the morning and evening for some nourishing ritual. | Start slow and choose one thing to do in the morning and in the evening to build back the practice of self-care and showing her body and mind that she is worth it and worth the time and effort. | Here setting actual time aside is important, even if it's just a few minutes. We want to create a habit toward self-love. We want to reprogram the mind from always putting her last to putting her first so she can be there for those she loves. |
| Mojo Mender | Daily reminders and exercises | Give herself permission to see herself. | Helps her gain confidence and self-worth. |

## Movement as Medicine

This yoga flow is designed to create space in your body, strength in your mind, and resilience in your spirit. The word *yoga* translates to "union," representing the beautiful connection between the self, your deeper essence, and your source of vitality. For the Silent Struggler, who often feels physically and emotionally depleted, this practice offers a gentle yet transformative pathway to healing. Through mindful movement and conscious breath, this flow helps shift your body and mind from a state of disconnection to one of reconnection and empowerment.

Each pose in this sequence is carefully selected to address the unique challenges faced by the Silent Struggler. For those experiencing chronic fatigue or hormonal imbalances, the flow incorporates gentle movements to stimulate circulation, improve lymphatic flow, and support hormonal balance. If your body feels fragile or weighed down by chronic pain, the poses help to release stored tension, increase flexibility, and build foundational strength without overwhelming your energy reserves.

On an emotional level, this yoga flow nurtures the nervous system, guiding it toward a parasympathetic state where true healing can occur. The Silent Struggler often carries unresolved emotions, stored in the body as physical tension, particularly in areas like the pelvic floor and the shoulders. By consciously creating space and flow in these areas, this practice encourages the release of those emotional burdens, helping you feel lighter and more aligned with your true self.

This yoga practice also focuses on cultivating self-compassion and trust—two vital elements for anyone rebuilding their health and identity. Each breath and movement invites you to listen to your body's needs, honor where you are in this moment, and find strength in your ability to adapt and grow. Over time, practicing this flow a few times a week can help you access a deeper connection with yourself, rebuild your energy, and regain the sense of vitality that is always within you.

Remember, this is not just a physical practice but a holistic one that supports your entire being—body, mind, and soul. Give yourself permission to lean into the process and watch how this flow helps you create a ripple effect of healing throughout your life.

## MORNING YOGA ROUTINE

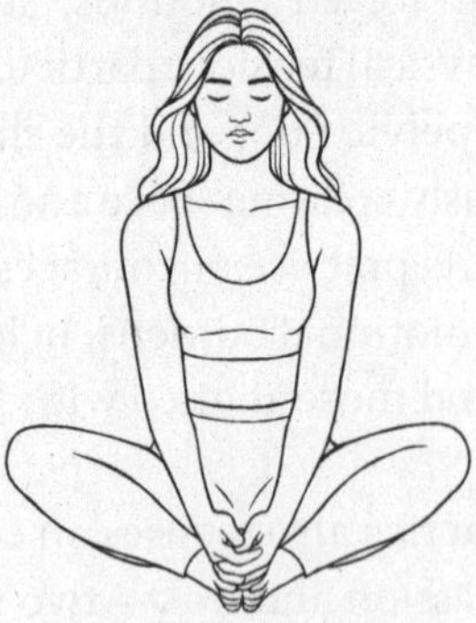

### Sufi Grind in Butterfly Pose

In a seated position, bring the soles of your feet together. Hold on to the feet and relax your shoulders. Begin to rotate over your hips in a clockwise direction. Inhale as you go forward and exhale as you come back. Circle in one direction for 1 minute and switch directions to counterclockwise for 1 more minute. Keep your eyes closed and focused at your brow point between your eyebrows.

### Cat Cow Pose (Marjaryasana and Bitilasana)

Come onto your hands and knees with knees hip width apart and your hands shoulder width apart. Inhale and lift your chin up, flexing the spine down into Cow and then exhale, bringing the chin back toward your chest and rounding your back into Cat. Feel the spaces between your vertebrae opening as you move through these postures. Continue for 1 to 3 minutes.

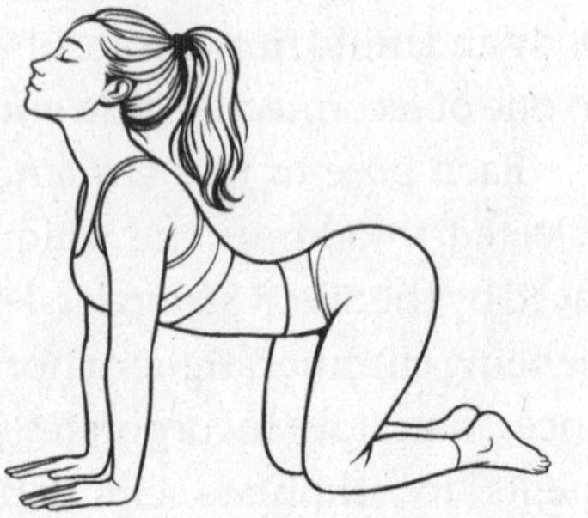

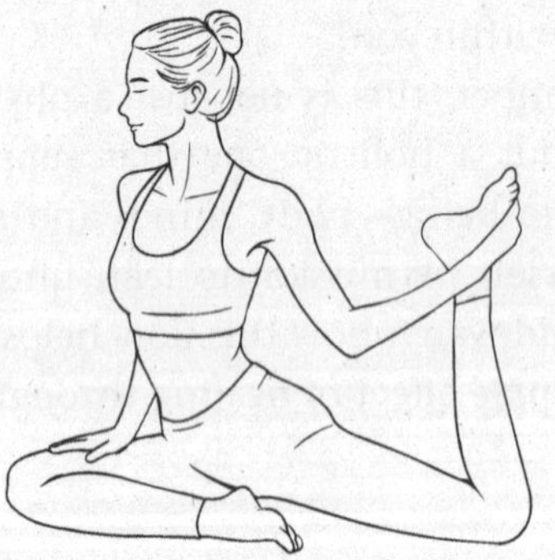

### Pigeon Pose (Eka Pada Rajakapotasana)

Bring one knee in front of you, keep the hips neutral, and make sure you are not over stretching your knee. Place your hands on the floor and lift your torso up, lengthening your spine and feel the stretch in your hips. Once you feel steady flex the back leg and grab a hold of your ankle. Breathe long and deep for 1 minute on one side and then switch sides.

### Child's Pose (Balasana)

Start your practice in child's pose with your knees apart, your forehead on the ground, and arms stretched overhead. Take a deep breath in through your nose to the count of 4, hold, and then let out an exhale through your mouth with a deep sigh to the count of 8. Repeat 3 times. While in this posture, create an intention for your practice.

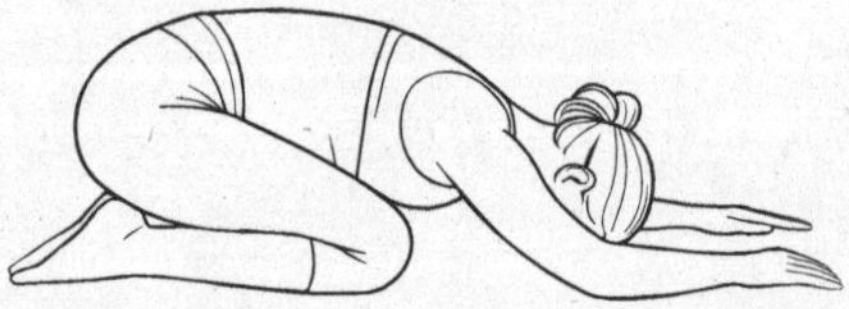

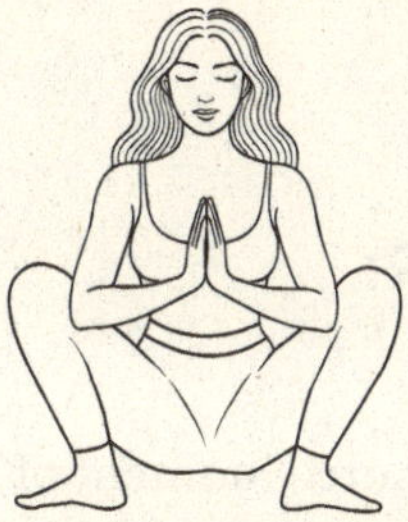

## Garland Pose (Malasana)

With your legs in a wide squat and feet pointing outward, bring your sit bones as close to the floor as possible. Bring the palms of your hands together in front of your heart. Relax your shoulders and in this position, begin Breath of Fire. Exhale through your nose while pumping your navel. Continue for 1 to 3 minutes.

## Warrior 2 to Archer Pose (Virabhadrasana II)

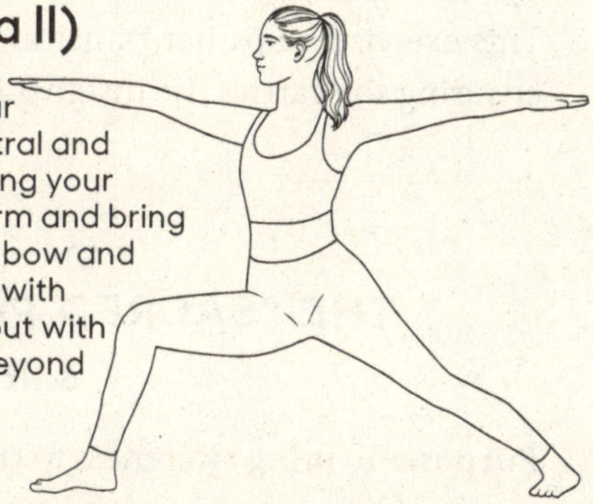

Come into a lunge position, keeping your front knee behind your toes. Rotate your back foot 45 degrees and keep your hips neutral and facing the front. Arms straight out and shoulders relaxed, keeping your gaze in front of you. After a few breaths here, take your back arm and bring it forward to meet the front and pull back as if you are pulling a bow and arrow. Your back elbow and upper arm are parallel to the floor with your hand close to your ear. Your front arm still points straight but with your fingers curled in and thumb sticking up. Keep your gaze beyond your thumb. Feel the strength in this posture. Breathe long and deep for 1 minute and then repeat on the other side.

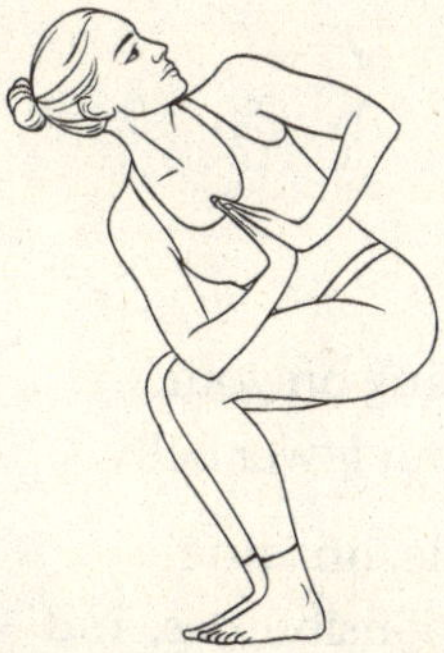

## Revolved Chair Pose (Parivrtta Utkatanasana)

Come to the front of your mat. With your legs together, find your grounding in your feet and sit back into chair pose. Bring your hands into prayer and twist to one side, allowing your elbow to settle on the outside of your knee. Breathe long and deep, and keep your gaze toward the sky. After a minute, repeat on the other side.

## Bridge Pose (Setu Bandha Sarvangasana)

Come lying on your back. Bend your knees and bring your heels close to your sit bones. You can grab hold of your ankles or place your hands on the floor and lift your pelvis to the sky, keeping your core engaged and your shoulder blades down and back. Keep your chin tucked in and breathe long and deep with your eyes closed. Continue for 1 minute.

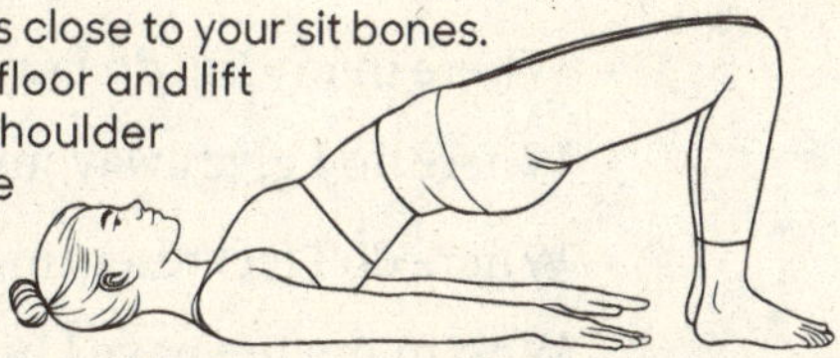

**Complete the set by lying on the ground in Savasana and internally chanting the mantra *I am, I am, I am*. Give yourself a few moments of gratitude for your body and all that is allowing you to experience in this lifetime.**

## POST-YOGA REFLECTION EXERCISE FOR THE SILENT STRUGGLER: RECLAIMING YOUR VOICE & NEEDS

For the Silent Struggler, movement alone is not enough—she needs a structured moment of reflection and intentional self-inquiry after her yoga practice. As a natural people-pleaser, she often prioritizes the needs of others over her own, leaving her depleted and resentful. This exercise helps her transition from movement to mental and emotional integration, ensuring she carries the insights from her practice into her daily life.

## EXERCISE: THE "SACRED PAUSE"—RELEASING OBLIGATION & RECLAIMING CHOICE

**Purpose:** To bring awareness to the unconscious ways the Silent Struggler says yes when she means **no**, and to reconnect her with what she truly desires.

**Time needed:** 5 to 10 minutes, right after yoga or meditation

**How to do it:**

1. **Find a comfortable seated position.** Keep your hands resting on your thighs or place one hand on your heart and the other on your lower belly.
2. **Close your eyes and take 3 deep breaths.** With each inhale, imagine filling yourself up; with each exhale, let go of the roles, responsibilities, and expectations that don't belong to you.
3. **Ask yourself:**
   - Where in my life do I say yes when I truly want to say no?
   - Where do I give away my time, energy, or emotions without being asked?
   - Where do I feel resentment in my body when I overextend myself?
   - Who in my life have I been prioritizing over my own needs?
4. **Journal (if possible):** Write down the **first 3 situations or relationships** that come to mind where you feel drained or obligated rather than inspired and fulfilled.

5. **Rewrite the story:** For each situation, write one sentence that reclaims your power, such as:
    - "I am allowed to disappoint others if it means staying true to myself."
    - "My worth is not determined by what I do for others."
    - "It is safe for me to receive as much as I give."

---

## INTEGRATION: THE ONE SMALL NO" PRACTICE

After completing the reflection, set an **intention to say one small no today**. It doesn't have to be drastic—just a single moment where you **pause** before responding and check in with yourself before automatically saying yes.

Examples of small nos:

- Not answering a text right away when someone asks for a favor.
- Choosing a meal you actually enjoy instead of what others want.
- Allowing yourself to leave a social event early when you feel drained.

Each small act of self-prioritization builds new neural pathways that reinforce self-worth and emotional balance, breaking the cycle of overgiving and depletion.

**Why it works:**

- Brings awareness to self-sacrificing habits in real time.
- Uses breath and stillness to process what comes up during movement.
- Creates an actionable step to reclaim personal space, voice, and emotional boundaries.
- Strengthens the nervous system's ability to pause before people-pleasing.

## Meals and More

To rebuild the physical form and fuel the mind with the energy and motivation needed for meaningful change, it's essential to focus on foods that are light, nutrient dense, and easily digestible. The Silent Struggler often faces challenges like chronic fatigue, inflammation, and gut sensitivity, which can make heavy or overly complex meals more taxing on the digestive system. When the body spends excessive energy on digestion, it has fewer resources to fuel hormone production, brain function, and emotional resilience. Simplifying meals not only aids digestion but also provides the body with the space it needs to heal and re-energize.

This identity often prioritizes the needs of others, both from a food perspective and in broader life contexts. Just as she may focus on "feeding" the emotional and physical needs of others before her own, she may struggle to see food as a form of self-care. The relationship we have with nourishment reflects the relationship we have with ourselves. For the Silent Struggler, this means unlearning the habit of always putting others first and beginning the transformation of prioritizing her own health and well-being. This shift doesn't happen overnight—it requires a change in belief systems and the creation of habits that remind her body and mind of the benefits of self-nourishment.

Starting with food as a foundation helps anchor this transformation. When she experiences how good her body feels after prioritizing nutrient-dense, digestible meals, it reinforces the belief that choosing herself is not selfish—it's necessary. Because this identity often struggles with immune responses, inflammation, and gut imbalances, eating simple, anti-inflammatory meals is key to reducing symptoms and improving overall health.

From the Ayurvedic perspective, the *kapha* constitution is often a helpful framework for the Silent Struggler. Kapha-focused meals emphasize light, warming, and easily digestible foods that boost metabolism, promote energy, and reduce the sluggishness that can accompany hormonal imbalances. Think of foods like gently steamed vegetables, warming spices such as ginger and cinnamon, and lighter proteins like lentils or white fish. Avoiding cold, heavy, or overly oily foods can also support improved digestion and energy flow.

Below is a chart you can follow to create an ideal day of meals. Each meal is designed to nourish your body while calming inflammation, supporting your digestion, and rebuilding your energy reserves. In the process of nourishing your physical body, you are also nourishing your emotional resilience and mental clarity, empowering you to show up for yourself in ways that feel sustainable and transformative.

## General Rules

1. Avoid heavy and oily foods with unhealthy oils in them.
2. Take time to have your meal and be intentional with every bite.
3. Put the utensils down between each bite and eat without distractions like screens.
4. Say a prayer or gratitude for the food and yourself before eating.
5. Eat a variety of seasonal whole foods.
6. Eat organic fruits and vegetables, especially those on the Dirty Dozen list, created by the Environmental Working Group, of produce items most contaminated with pesticides.
7. Avoid genetically modified ingredients.

The following foods will help you re-establish a relationship with your digestion, metabolism, and energy. When your digestion feels vital, so do your hormones. It is hard to feel motivated in life when you feel heavy in the belly, energetically and physically. Creating conscious habits around food choices reduces inflammation and gives room for your body and mind to feel strong and healthy.

| FOODS TO AVOID | FOODS TO INCLUDE |
|---|---|
| **Grains:**<br>Wheat | **Grains:**<br>Buckwheat<br>Millet<br>Barley<br>Rice |
| **Vegetables:** Any that are too sweet and very sour<br>Potatoes<br>Tomatoes<br>Water chestnuts | **Vegetables:** Most veggies work; eating them steamed is preferred, but raw is also good<br>Leafy greens<br>Seed vegetables, such as bell peppers<br>Peppers |
| **Fruits:** Avoid any too sweet or sour | **Fruits:**<br>Plums<br>Apples<br>Apricots<br>Cranberries<br>Mangoes<br>Peaches<br>Pears<br>Pomegranates |
| **Dairy/Fish/Meat:**<br>Anything fried<br>Cow milk | **Dairy/Fish/Meat:**<br>Chicken<br>Eggs<br>Small amounts of ghee<br>Goat milk |
| **Legumes:**<br>Black lentils<br>Kidney beans<br>Soybeans | **Legumes:**<br>Black beans<br>Mung beans<br>Pinto beans<br>Red lentils |
| **Nuts/Seeds/Oils:** Avoid most nuts and oils | **Nuts/Seeds/Oils:**<br>Sunflower seeds<br>Pumpkin seeds<br>Almond oil |

# Breakfast

Breakfast can be light for this constitution, like a green smoothie in the warmer months. This constitution does well with intermittent fasting and not eating until midmorning or lunch. In the fasting window, one can have a nourishing elixir with warming spices and some ghee.

---

## Warming Chai

1 cup filtered water
A few cardamom pods
A few cloves
½ teaspoon minced fresh ginger root
A few crushed peppercorns
1 cinnamon stick
1 teaspoon black tea (optional)
Milk of your choice, for serving
Ground cinnamon (optional)
Honey (optional)

Place all the ingredients into a pot and boil until the water is down to half. Strain into a cup and add your choice of warm alternative milk. Sprinkle some cinnamon on top and add some honey for sweetness.

---

## Red Lentil Pancakes

1 cup red lentils, soaked overnight
½ teaspoon cumin powder
½ teaspoon coriander powder
½ teaspoon curry powder
½ teaspoon paprika
½ teaspoon garam masala
1 clove garlic, finely chopped
1 slice ginger, finely chopped
1¼ cups filtered water
½ teaspoon Celtic sea salt
2 teaspoons chickpea flour
1 tablespoon coconut oil, avocado oil, or ghee
1 bunch cilantro, chopped (optional)
Vegan cream or yogurt, for serving

Place all the ingredients except the cilantro in a blender and blend until smooth, like pancake batter. Oil a cast-iron pan with coconut or avocado oil, or ghee. Pour the batter into the pan as you would a pancake or crepe and cook each side for about 2 minutes on medium-low heat. You can top with some cilantro or other sauteed vegetables, like zucchini, and a vegan cream or yogurt.

# Lunch

## Leafy Greens and Chickpea Salad

1 tablespoon ghee, divided
1 small white onion, chopped into small pieces
A few slices ginger, chopped
3 to 4 cloves chopped garlic, divided
1 teaspoon cumin
1 teaspoon coriander
1 teaspoon garam masala
1 teaspoon curry powder
1 teaspoon Celtic sea salt, or more, to taste
One 13.5-ounce (400 ml) can organic chickpeas
One 13.5-ounce (400 ml) can coconut milk
1 cup chopped dandelion greens
1 cup chopped spinach
1 cup chopped Swiss chard
Black pepper, to taste
Olive oil and lemon juice, for serving (optional)

Add your ghee and onions into a pot. When the onion becomes translucent, add in the ginger and half of the garlic. Cook for a few minutes on medium-low heat. Add in the spices and stir well. Add in the chickpeas and coconut milk and let simmer for about 10 to 15 minutes, until they look creamy and well cooked. In a separate pan, add some ghee and garlic, and add in all the chopped greens with some salt and pepper to taste. On your plate you can use the greens as a bed for the curried chickpeas. I like to add some olive oil and a little lemon juice to the greens as well.

# Dinner

## Kitchari

1 to 2 tablespoons ghee
1 teaspoon shredded ginger
1 teaspoon fennel seeds
2 teaspoons cumin powder
1 teaspoon coriander powder
1 teaspoon turmeric
½ teaspoon paprika
1 teaspoon sea salt
1 cup yellow or red lentils, or yellow split peas
½ cup basmati rice
5 to 6 cups filtered water, or 4 cups vegetable broth and 2 cups filtered water
1 head broccoli, chopped
1 medium zucchini, shredded
1 bunch chopped spinach
1 bunch chopped cilantro

Stir the ghee, ginger, and fennel seeds in a pot. After about 30 seconds, add in the rest of the spices and stir. Cook for another 30 seconds. Add in the lentils, rice, and water and simmer for 35 to 40 minutes, until the rice and lentils become soft. Add in the chopped broccoli and cover for another 5 minutes. Turn off the heat and add in the zucchini, spinach, and cilantro.

## Herbs: Medicine from the Earth

The herbs I have chosen here are to build strength in the reproductive/hormonal system, rejuvenate the thyroid, and support the immune system. The combination of these can reset and give a jump start to your vitality while supporting the needs of your hormones. Speak to your functional physician about these options and how you can incorporate them into your life.

| NAME OF HERB | ACTIONS |
|---|---|
| *Shatavari* (*Asparagus racemosus*)—translates to "she who possesses a thousand husbands"—that's a lot of strength one needs to deal with all of that! | Helps to rejuvenate the blood and female organs, strengthens the immune system and mucous membranes, helping to strengthen the bladder and vaginal area. It also supports your capacity to manage stress. You can use it in a powdered form and mix it with ghee or in a capsule. |
| Rhodiola (golden root) | Helps build stamina, strength, energy, and vitality while alleviating mental overwhelm. Increases resistance toward mental and physical stress. May also support more insulin sensitivity. |
| Shilajit | Contains fulvic acid, so while it supports your gut microbiome, it also promotes strength, longevity, and even libido. |
| *Astragalus membranaceus* | Chinese herb used as an energy tonic. It increases the strength of your life force, your prana and chi. |
| Guggal (*Commiphora mukul*) | In conjunction with an adaptogen, helps to support regulation of your thyroid system. Helps to increase energy and metabolism while supporting communication in the reproductive system. |
| Black cohosh (*Cimicifuga racemosa*) | Can be used in conjunction with chaste berry to balance the estrogen and progesterone levels. Estrogenic in nature, this can help create symptom relief for many suffering with low-estrogen symptoms and depletion. |
| Rosmarinic acid | Calming effect on the immune system and acts as an anti-inflammatory agent. By reducing inflammation, you remove the noise around the cells, leaving room for your hormones to communicate as needed. |

## Vitamins and Minerals

For the Silent Struggler, navigating life while feeling depleted often becomes the norm, but it doesn't have to be. Vitamins and minerals play a foundational role in restoring the body's vitality and supporting the hormones that regulate energy, mood, and overall health. When the body is under chronic stress or dealing with emotional strain, the Silent Struggler's reserves of essential nutrients are often the first to be depleted. These nutrients, like magnesium and B vitamins, are crucial for hormone production, immune function, and energy metabolism.

Without adequate levels of these key vitamins and minerals, the body struggles to perform basic repair and recovery tasks, leading to symptoms such as fatigue, brain fog, weakened immunity, and hormonal imbalances. For women in this state, nourishing the body with the right micronutrients can act as the first step toward rebuilding strength and creating resilience.

Think of these nutrients as tools for rebuilding a strong foundation. They support the body's natural detoxification pathways, help regulate stress hormones like cortisol, and contribute to a steady mood and clearer thinking. For the Silent Struggler, prioritizing a nutrient-dense diet, targeted supplementation (under the guidance of a practitioner), and reducing nutrient-depleting habits like overreliance on caffeine or processed foods can bring profound improvements.

Restoring your body's nutritional reserves is an act of self-care that reinforces your strength and supports the healing journey ahead. By giving your body what it needs, you can begin to shed the weight of depletion and step into a life of more energy, balance, and joy.

| NAME | ACTIONS |
|---|---|
| Selenium | Supports production of thyroid hormone and immune system, and prevents cell damage. |
| Tyrosine or L-tyrosine | Precursor to dopamine, the neurotransmitter needed for motivation. |
| B complex | Needed for energy and resilience in the body. |
| Vitamin C | For immune and adrenal support. |
| Vitamin D | Needed for immunity, hormones, and so much more! |
| *Bifidobacterium lactis*<br>*Lactobacillus salivarius* | Shown to create healthy flora of hormonal balance, energy, and reproductive health, especially when used with inulin as a prebiotic to activate them. |
| Amino acids | Building blocks and foundational to vitality and health. |
| Magnesium glycinate | Can help in energy production, reduce PMS symptoms, relieve cramping, and support the thyroid and immune systems. |

## Mindset: I Am Worthy

Reprogramming self-doubt into self-respect is a transformative journey that requires daily intention and consistent practice. Tools like chanting and singing are powerful allies on this path. Not only do these practices increase vagal tone—helping your mind and body shift into a state of calm and regulation—but they also provide a space to plant seeds of new, empowering beliefs. Through sound and repetition, you can begin to reinforce your sense of self-worth and recognize the importance of prioritizing yourself.

For many women, putting themselves first feels unnatural, even uncomfortable. Generations of conditioning have tied our sense of value to acts of service for others, leaving little room to focus on our own needs. Undoing this programming is no small task, but it begins with simple, intentional steps that gradually move you closer to your true self. This process isn't about rejecting service to others but redefining it to include service to yourself—because when you are well, everyone benefits.

One way to start this shift is by dedicating time each day to honor your brilliance and unique value. Writing a letter to your younger self can be a deeply healing exercise and one that can start to heal the deep layers of beliefs. Reflect on what you wish she had known, the guidance you would have given her, and the dreams you hope she holds on to. Be selfish in your reflections. Be courageous in your words. And be committed to honoring her journey, as it has shaped the woman you are today.

By creating space for these moments of reflection and self-respect, you begin to establish healthy boundaries that protect your energy and allow you to focus on your health and happiness. Below is a meditation designed to awaken the inner goddess within you—the part of you that is ready to receive the gifts the universe has been waiting to offer. Through this practice, you can step into a space of deserving, courage, and unwavering commitment to your journey.

*Sit in a comfortable seat. Feel your sit bones anchored to the ground. Bring your left hand to your heart center and your right hand to just above your navel, your solar plexus. Close your eyes. Focus your eyes above, in between your eyebrows, the seat of your intuition and ability to see the truth. Begin to take a deep breath in through your nose while expanding your belly to the count of 5, pause to the count of 5, and exhale through the nose, bringing your belly back to your spine and letting it all go to the count of 10, and pause for the count of 5. As you continue to breathe in your inner mind, begin to repeat* Shakti, *meaning "feminine power." Continue to silently chant this mantra as you breathe deeply, consciously letting go of the old patterns and beliefs, inviting nourishment and vitality through your breath, and declaring your power all at once. Finish it off by chanting the mantra* So hum, *meaning, "I am." Chant loud and unapologetically! Or put on a good tune you love and sing your heart out!*

Do this meditation for however long life permits. You can start with just a few minutes and gradually increase your time. You may notice after a few days, you start to crave the feeling of connection you get from sitting with yourself.

## Morning/Evening Rituals of Bliss

This section is one of the most essential because it focuses on cultivating the habits of self-care—a foundation for lasting healing. For the Silent Struggler, these rituals are more than just acts of physical care; they are an invitation to reconnect with yourself, acknowledge your needs, and nurture your emotional and mental well-being. When you've spent years prioritizing others, neglecting your health, or feeling disconnected from your true self, these rituals offer a safe space to rebuild, little by little.

The Silent Struggler often feels depleted and unseen, juggling the weight of her responsibilities while quietly carrying unspoken pain. For her, these rituals are vital because they serve as gentle reminders that she is worthy of care and attention—not just from others, but from herself. Incorporating daily practices is like planting seeds of self-compassion and self-respect, allowing them to grow into lasting habits that strengthen her body, mind, and spirit.

Each ritual is designed to support holistic health. On a physical level, they improve circulation, digestion, and hormonal balance. Emotionally, they help to release stored stress and tension while creating space for joy and calm. Mentally, these habits encourage presence, grounding, and a sense of control amid life's chaos. They also work as anchors during moments of overwhelm, providing structure and consistency when everything else feels unsteady.

These rituals are particularly important for the Silent Struggler, because they are acts of reclaiming power and self-worth. They offer a way to shift the narrative from "I'm not enough" to "I deserve this time for me." Simple acts like mindful breathing, enjoying a warm herbal tea, or journaling about your feelings create powerful ripples of healing. Over time, these small moments accumulate into a larger sense of resilience and inner strength.

Below are some nourishing rituals you can choose from to support your mental, emotional, and physical health. Start with just one or two, and as they become part of your routine, you can add more. Remember, this is your time to invest in yourself—guilt-free and with the knowledge that caring for yourself will help you show up more fully in all areas of your life.

# Morning

1. Essential oil of rosemary: As soon as you wake up, smell this essential oil to wake up your senses. It lowers stress while improving alertness.
2. Morning drink: Make one of these drinks to jump start your digestion and nourish your nervous system.
   - Juice some ginger and lime and blend with some basil. Add a pinch of salt and enjoy your morning drink.
   - If you prefer a warmer drink, you can boil a teaspoon of fennel seeds and some cardamom pods in a cup of water; strain and enjoy.
3. Morning affirmation: Before getting up, the goal is to not give your mind the opportunity to remind you of all you need to do, must do, and can't do. We are going to choose to declare your awesomeness right away. Below are some examples . . .

   "I choose to say yes to joy."
   "My body is working for me, not against me."
   "I deserve abundance."
   "I am worthy."
   "I choose ease."

## Evening

1. Gift yourself with time for yourself to journal. Below are some prompts that can help you . . .
   - List 3 things you did for yourself that day.
   - List what didn't work for you that day.
   - Where did you show up as your true self, and where did you show up as your conditioned self?
   - Were there certain environments and certain people that pulled you back into old habits and patterns?
   - What nourished you today, and what depleted you?
2. Massage Marma Heart Point (*hridaya*) with essential oil of rose: This oil helps to calm the heart and nourishes the soul. Place a few drops on your sternum and massage in a circular motion while lying down.
3. Navel oiling: According to Ayurveda, navel oiling can help the body and mind. The navel is where 72,000 nerve endings come together to communicate with the rest of the body, supporting your hormones and nervous system.

### Rebuilding Connection Through Boundaries & Support—Relationship Edition

The Silent Struggler often carries her relationships on her shoulders, silently absorbing the needs, emotions, and expectations of those around her. She is the one everyone leans on, but rarely does she allow herself to lean back. This dynamic creates silent resentment, not because she does not love those around her, but because she feels unseen, unheard, and unsupported. Healing for the Silent Struggler is about transforming relationships from obligation into mutual care and respect. These practices will help her break the cycle of overgiving, build emotional safety, and allow her to receive love and support in return.

## 1. THE "I MATTER TOO" PRACTICE—HEALING THE OVERGIVING PATTERN

The Silent Struggler is often the first to say yes and the last to consider her own needs. This exercise helps her acknowledge her own importance in relationships by recognizing the imbalance of giving and receiving.

### Practice for Self-Reflection

*(5 minutes before making a decision in a relationship)*

1. Before saying yes to a request or responsibility, pause and ask yourself:
    - "Am I saying yes because I want to, or because I feel obligated?"
    - "What would I need in return to feel balanced in this exchange?"
    - "What happens when I prioritize my needs as much as others'?"
2. Close your eyes, place a hand on your heart, and take 3 deep breaths. Imagine yourself receiving instead of giving.
3. If saying yes feels draining or misaligned, practice saying:
    - "I need to think about that before committing."
    - "I can't take that on right now, but I appreciate you asking."
    - "I would love to help, but I need support in return."

**Why it works:**

- Interrupts automatic overgiving.
- Teaches the Silent Struggler to advocate for herself in relationships.
- Prevents silent resentment from building up.

## 2. THE "MUTUAL CARE CHECK-IN"— RESTORING BALANCE IN RELATIONSHIPS

The Silent Struggler often assumes responsibility for emotional labor, carrying the weight of organizing, remembering, and emotionally supporting her partner and family. This check-in creates balance by making sure both partners are heard, seen, and supported.

### Couple's Exercise: A Weekly Relationship Reset
*(15 minutes, once a week)*

1. Each partner gets 5 minutes to share what they need support with. The other listens without offering advice or problem-solving.
2. Each partner asks the other:
    - "What's something I can take off your plate this week?"
    - "How can I emotionally support you right now?"
    - "What is one thing you wish I acknowledged more?"
3. Silent Struggler's Challenge:
    - Ask for something that feels uncomfortable to receive.
    - Notice the urge to deflect or say, "I'm fine."
    - Let yourself be cared for.

**Why it works:**

- Stops the Silent Struggler from carrying all emotional labor alone.
- Encourages her partner to actively participate in the relationship.
- Builds a habit of mutual care.

## 3. "REWRITING THE STORY"— A PRACTICE FOR RELEASING OLD RELATIONSHIP PATTERNS

Many Silent Strugglers carry a deeply ingrained belief that they must be the strong one, or else relationships will fall apart. This belief keeps them stuck in cycles of overresponsibility and burnout.

### Journaling Exercise

*(use when resentment or exhaustion arises in relationships)*

1. Write down the belief that keeps you stuck. (Examples: "I have to do everything, or it won't get done." "If I don't take care of them, they won't love me." "My needs don't matter.")
2. Reflect on where this belief came from.
   - Did you watch your mother overgive in relationships?
   - Was love in your childhood home given conditionally?
   - Did you learn that your needs were secondary?
3. Reframe the belief into an empowering statement.
   - *Old belief:* "If I say no, people will leave."
   - *New belief:* "I am loved and valued for who I am, not just what I do for others."

**Why it works:**

- Helps break free from inherited relationship patterns.
- Encourages self-compassion.
- Releases the guilt around asking for support.

## 4. "TOUCH WITHOUT OBLIGATION"— A PRACTICE TO HEAL INTIMACY

For many Silent Strugglers, exhaustion leads to emotional and physical disconnection from their partners. Affection starts to feel like another demand rather than a source of comfort. This practice restores intimacy without pressure.

### Couple's Exercise: The 10-Minute Hold

*(use daily or when feeling emotionally distant)*

1. Sit or lie down facing each other.
2. One partner places their hand over the other's heart. Hold eye contact without speaking.
3. Breathe together for 2 to 3 minutes, synchronizing breath.
4. The Silent Struggler allows herself to receive touch without needing to give back immediately.
5. After 10 minutes, reflect:
   - How did it feel to receive without giving?
   - What emotions arose?
   - How does your body feel compared to before?

**Why it works:**

- Restores connection without pressure.
- Helps the Silent Struggler feel safe in receiving love.
- Allows intimacy to feel nourishing rather than exhausting.

## 5. THE "PERMISSION TO NEED" MEDITATION—HEALING THE FEAR OF ASKING FOR SUPPORT

One of the biggest challenges for the Silent Struggler is admitting she needs help, care, or rest. This guided visualization helps her release the guilt around receiving.

### Guided Meditation:
### *(5 to 7 minutes before bed)*

1. Close your eyes and place both hands on your chest.
2. Breathe deeply, inhaling through the nose, exhaling slowly through the mouth.
3. Imagine yourself as a young girl, exhausted and needing comfort.
4. Visualize your adult self stepping forward and saying:
   - "You don't have to carry this alone."
   - "You are allowed to rest."
   - "You are loved even when you're not doing."
5. Breathe in acceptance, exhale guilt.
6. End by whispering: "I give myself permission to receive."

**Why it works:**

- Releases the subconscious belief that needing support is weak.
- Teaches the Silent Struggler's nervous system to feel safe in rest.
- Builds emotional self-compassion.

The Silent Struggler's journey is not about changing who she is—it's about learning that she is worthy of receiving as much love as she gives.

CHAPTER 11

# Breaking the Cycle of Perfect

## Plan C: Rewriting the Rules of Perfect with the HER Method

The focus of this plan is to help remove all the obstacles to healing—whether they are toxic thoughts, harmful environments, inflammatory foods, hormone disruptors, or even relationships that drain your energy. For women dealing with conditions like fibroids, cysts, endometriosis, polycystic ovarian syndrome (PCOS), or hormonal acne, the importance of detoxifying the physical, emotional, and mental bodies cannot be overstated. These conditions are often a manifestation of deeper imbalances, not just in the hormones themselves but in the environments and patterns that have shaped their lives.

The Perfectionist with a Price, in particular, may find herself especially prone to these conditions due to the chronic stress and pressure she places on herself to meet unattainable standards. The drive to excel at all costs can lead to inflammation, hormonal imbalances, and even the stagnation of energy in the body—all of which can exacerbate these health challenges. Healing for the Perfectionist with a Price requires more than just treating the physical symptoms; it calls for a holistic approach that addresses the root causes, including the mental clutter, emotional baggage, and toxic narratives that have been carried for too long.

By learning to detox not just her body but also her mind and spirit, the Perfectionist can begin to release the patterns that have kept her stuck in cycles of perfectionism and self-criticism. This process involves creating space for rest, reflection, and nourishment—things that may feel unfamiliar or even indulgent to her. Yet, these are the very acts that allow her body to heal, her hormones to rebalance, and her mind to find peace. Letting go of the need to control every outcome and embracing a mindset of surrender and self-compassion are vital steps in this journey.

Through detoxification and intentional healing practices, women with these conditions—and particularly those who identify as Perfectionists—can transform their health and well-being. They can create a new narrative, one that prioritizes their health, allows for imperfection, and celebrates their worth, not for what they do but for who they are. This path of healing is not just about managing symptoms; it's about reclaiming their vitality and stepping into a life of balance and freedom.

| 5M MODEL | TYPE | CONSIDERATIONS | THE WHY |
|---|---|---|---|
| Movement | Yoga—Ashtanga, Hatha<br>Hiking<br>High-intensity interval training and/or low-intensity interval training | For this identity, it's important to choose movement that will get her moving and sweating. It is also important for her to reconnect with her body and build self-confidence and self-trust through getting to know her body and even its limits. Moving the lymphatic system here is also key. It is the cleanup system in the body and needs movement for activation. | Sweating is a pathway of elimination for toxins. Movement like this gives us access to feel-good hormones and neurotransmitters, and brain-derived neurotropic factor, a key ingredient for a healthy relationship with self. The more confident a woman feels in her body, the more confident she feels in making choices that help her let go of the vices, people, and circumstances that don't support her. |
| Meals and Nutrition | Liver-friendly foods incorporated daily<br>Fasting practices<br>Detoxing and nourishing foods that cool down the heat of inflammation | Because this identity has often tried it all, it is important to simplify and clear the clutter. Choose meals that are simple, detoxing, and anti-inflammatory. | If the digestive system is inflamed, it makes it harder to detox the toxins, excess hormones from the environment, and even the mind/emotions. By simplifying the diet and incorporating fasting, you create space beyond the chaos. |

| | | | |
|---|---|---|---|
| Mindset | Time in nature<br>Breathwork | Find time to breathe, especially fresh air from nature. Time in nature and even a little time at home, at work, or in the car to tune in to your breath can help bring you back into your body, reconnecting to yourself and the source of life, oxygen. | Pathogens don't like oxygen. They thrive in anaerobic (low-oxygen) environments. Change your environment, change your life. Through breath you not only create an oxygenated environment filled with prana, your life force, you are consciously detoxing and removing toxins out of your body. |
| Morning/ Evening Rituals | Humming breath<br>Marma points<br>Clearing and letting go | Rituals that bring your awareness to the present moment while reminding you that you are beautiful as you are. Give yourself permission to let go and believe in your own potential. | Part of detoxing our internal environment is to detox the external. Paying attention to where you put your focus in the morning and before bed, from the thoughts you are having to the products you are applying all will impact your day and your health. |
| Mojo Mender | Exercises and practices | Daily reminders that give you time to reflect. | Helps you see you are enough as you are. |

## Movement as Medicine

The following yoga postures offer more than just physical benefits—they serve as a powerful practice for cleansing the body and releasing the mental and emotional grip of perfectionism. By incorporating breathwork alongside movement, these postures help to flush toxins from your body while also creating a sense of spaciousness in both your body and mind. This spaciousness is crucial for the Perfectionist, who often feels weighed down by the need to control and achieve in every area of life.

Stretching the body through these postures not only helps to release physical tension but also mirrors the release of mental tension, creating a gateway to let go of the rigid attachment to perfection. As you move through these postures, you may notice that the same energy you once channeled into striving for flawlessness can now be redirected into building strength, flow, and resilience.

The Perfectionist archetype often has a tendency to ignore the body's cues in favor of outward appearances or external achievements. These yoga postures encourage a reconnection to your body's innate wisdom, helping you to tune in to what it truly needs. The focus here is on stimulating the lymphatic system to encourage detoxification, strengthening the core to build inner and outer stability, and cultivating a sense of confidence that comes from within rather than from external validation.

This practice becomes a metaphor for life—showing you that it's okay to stumble, to wobble, and to find your balance again. Through movement, you learn to trust the process and embrace imperfection, which is where true healing begins. With consistent practice, you'll notice not only improvements in your physical health but also a shift in your mindset, empowering you to shed the unrealistic expectations you've placed on yourself.

This journey is about more than just yoga; it's about reclaiming your body, your mind, and your spirit from the stranglehold of perfectionism. It's a practice of stepping into your power and honoring yourself, just as you are, while allowing space for growth, healing, and joy.

## MORNING YOGA ROUTINE

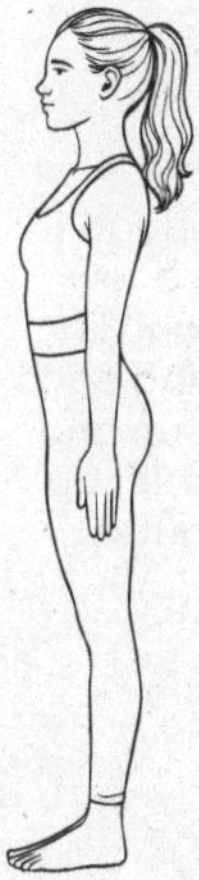

### Mountain Pose (Tadasana)

Come standing with your feet rooted to the ground and hip distance apart. Lift the inner arches of your feet up and root down on all four corners of your feet. Draw your inner thighs back, lengthen your torso, broaden the upper back, and draw your belly in and up. Draw your shoulder blades down your back and broaden your collar bones. Arms straight and palms facing forward, and have your chin parallel to the floor. Soften your gaze and breathe long and deep.

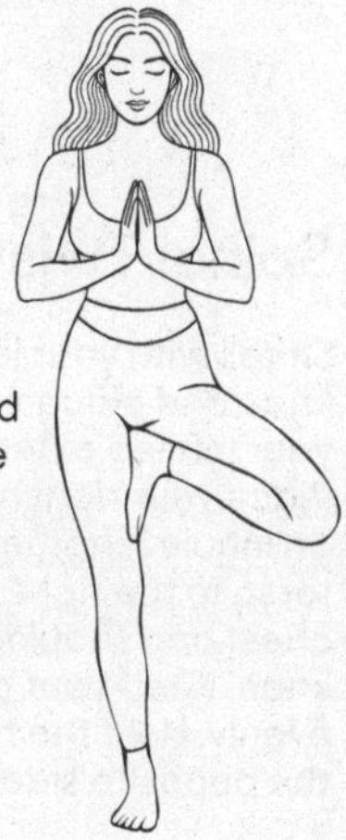

### Tree Pose with Breath of Fire (Vrksasana)

Come standing on both feet hip width apart. Put a bit more weight on one foot, and when you feel steady on that foot, lift the other foot and bring the sole to touch the standing leg's inner thigh while keeping the hips neutral. Bring your hands into prayer and find a spot on the floor you can focus on for balance and begin Breath of Fire. Passively inhale and actively exhale through the nose while pumping your . navel. Continue for 1 to 3 minutes. Repeat on the other side.

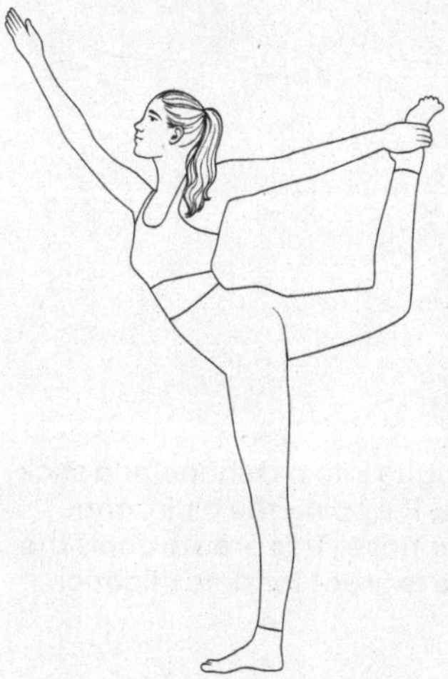

### Dancer's Pose (Natarajasana)

Steady yourself on one foot. Lift the other leg as you bring the same hand back to grab the inner part of the foot of the lifted leg. Bring the opposite arm in front of you for balance. Relax your shoulders and create neutrality in your hips. Don't forget to breathe and tap into your inner dancer! Repeat on the opposite side.

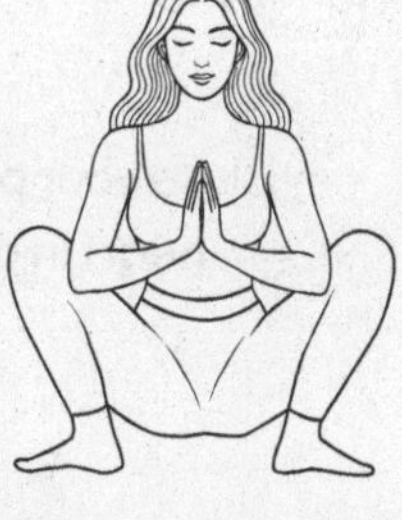

### Garland Pose (Malasana)

With your legs in a wide squat and feet pointing outward, bring your sit bones as close to the floor as possible. Bring the palms of your hands together in front of your heart. Relax your shoulders and in this position, begin Breath of Fire. Exhale through your nose while pumping your navel. Continue for 1 to 3 minutes.

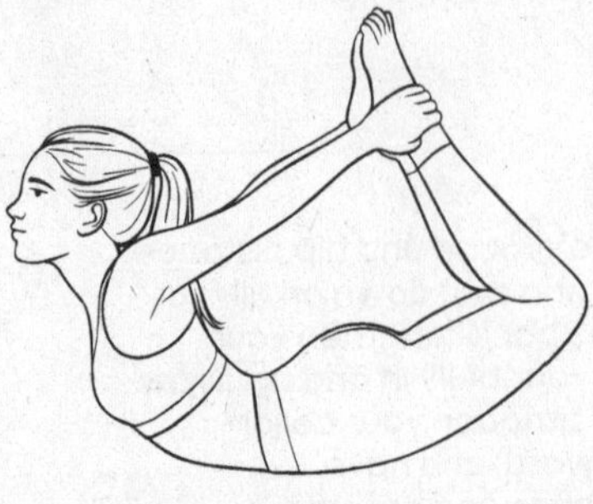

## Bow Pose (Dhanurasana)

Come lying on your belly and place your forehead to the ground with your arms by your side. Take a few deep breaths and begin to bend your knees and lift your lower legs toward your sit bones, grabbing each ankle with your hands and pulling your chest up and open. Keep your chin tucked in. On the inhale, lift up and on the exhale relax. Repeat for 1 to 3 minutes.

## Spinal Twist (Ardha Matsyendrasana)

Sit tall with your legs extended in front of you, then bend your right knee and place your right foot to the outside of your left thigh. Keep your left leg extended or bend it so the heel rests near your right hip. Place your right hand on the floor just behind you for support, and on an inhale lengthen through your spine. As you exhale, gently twist your torso to the right, starting from your belly and moving up through your chest and shoulders. Bring your left elbow to the outside of your right knee. Keep your gaze over your right shoulder, breathing deeply and evenly. Hold the twist for 1 minute, then slowly release and repeat on the opposite side.

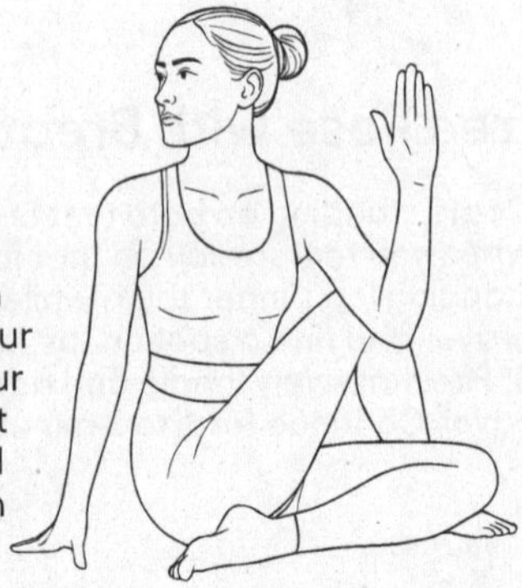

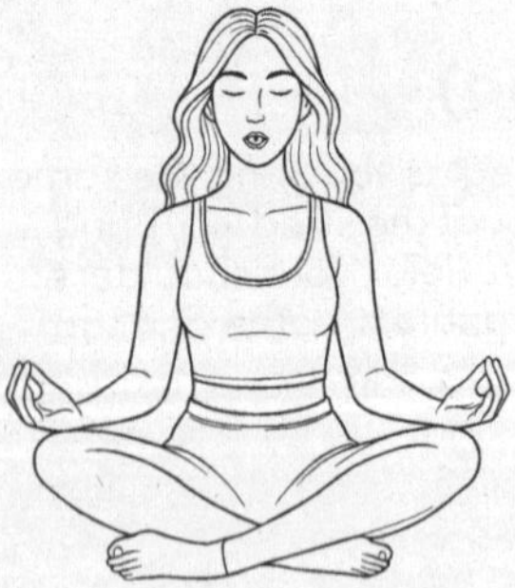

## Sitali Pranayama

Sit in a comfortable position. Curl your tongue into a U shape and stick it out slightly. Inhale through the tongue as if sipping the air in, and close your mouth and exhale through your nose. This breath cools the body down (amazing for hot flashes!) and is great for detoxification.

**Close your practice with a moment of silence while you place your hands over your heart in gratitude for your life, your health, and your commitment to yourself.**

## POST-YOGA REFLECTION EXERCISE FOR THE PERFECTIONIST WITH A PRICE: RELEASING THE MASK & EMBRACING AUTHENTIC CONNECTION

For the Perfectionist with a Price, movement is often about control—an attempt to sculpt the body, discipline the mind, or force herself into a version of perfection that feels "worthy" of love and success. After yoga, she needs a practice that shifts her from control to surrender and helps her reflect on how perfectionism impacts her ability to connect with herself authentically.

## EXERCISE: "THE MIRROR OF ENOUGHNESS"— SEEING YOURSELF CLEARLY

**Purpose:** To help you recognize where perfectionism is keeping you from genuine self-acceptance and inner peace.

**Time needed:** 5 to 10 minutes after yoga

**How to do it:**

1. **Find a comfortable seated position** (cross-legged or with back supported).
2. **Place one hand on your heart and one hand on your belly.** Close your eyes and take slow, deep breaths. With each inhale, feel your body expand; with each exhale, let go of tension in your face, jaw, and shoulders.
3. **Ask yourself:**
    - Where in my life do I feel like I have to "perform" or be perfect to feel worthy?
    - What part of myself do I keep hidden because I think it's "not enough" or "too much"?
    - What would change if I released the need to prove myself and embraced being exactly who I am?
    - What is one thing I can do today that allows me to show up as I am, without perfection?

4. **Write it down (if possible):** Jot down one or two ways perfectionism has kept you from fully embracing yourself.
5. **Release-the-Mask Visualization:**
   - Picture yourself wearing a mask—the mask of perfection, control, or having it all together.
   - As you exhale, imagine slowly peeling the mask away, feeling the tension in your body release as you let go of the need to be anything other than yourself.
   - See your reflection in your mind's eye, not as a version to fix or improve, but as a person who is already whole.
   - Breathe into this feeling of freedom and relief as you allow yourself to be fully seen by yourself.

---

## INTEGRATION: "PERMISSION TO BE SEEN" PRACTICE

For the next 24 hours, challenge yourself to let go of 1 percent of perfectionism in a real-world situation.

- Leave one typo in a text or e-mail without double-checking.
- Allow yourself to be "unpolished" in a conversation and speak freely.
- Let yourself be seen in an unguarded moment—without adjusting, perfecting, or filtering.
- Say, "I don't know" when you don't have the answer instead of pretending you do.

These micro moments rewire your brain to accept that imperfection doesn't equal failure—it leads to deeper self-acceptance.

**Why it works:**

- Interrupts the performance cycle by helping the Perfectionist with a Price reflect on where she hides herself.
- Uses visualization to create a safe, internal experience of being vulnerable before doing it in real life.
- Breaks the all-or-nothing mindset by allowing small, daily steps toward authenticity.

## Meals and More

The Perfectionist often approaches life with a "do more, achieve more" mindset, which can extend to her relationship with food and her body. This drive for perfection may lead to rigid meal schedules, snacking throughout the day, or focusing too heavily on rigid dietary rules, leaving little room for her body to naturally reset and heal. Giving the body a break between meals is an essential practice for creating space—not just for digestion, but for healing and restoration on a cellular level.

Fasting is not about deprivation but about connection. For the Perfectionist, it offers an opportunity to step away from the constant striving and listen to the innate healing intelligence within. It is a chance to clear the clutter—physical, mental, and emotional—that has been weighing her down and awakening her body's natural potential to repair and rejuvenate. Fasting also provides a metaphorical and literal pause, allowing her to reflect on whether the constant hustle is serving her highest good or simply feeding the narrative of perfectionism.

From an Ayurvedic perspective, this approach focuses on clearing and pacifying the *pitta* dosha, which governs fire and transformation. Pitta imbalances can show up as inflammation, irritability, and burnout—common experiences for the Perfectionist. By addressing inflammation and eliminating ama (toxins) from the body, the Perfectionist can release not just physical burdens but also the emotional residue tied to her relentless pursuit of perfection.

This seven-day plan incorporates a mono-diet kitchari fast, a traditional Ayurvedic practice that simplifies digestion while providing nourishment. Kitchari, made from mung beans, rice, and spices, is gentle on the digestive system, allowing the body to redirect energy toward detoxification and healing. For the Perfectionist, who is accustomed to overloading her schedule and her mind, this practice introduces a sense of simplicity and calm, creating space for self-reflection and healing.

Fasting also has profound benefits for the mind. It activates clarity, reduces mental fog, and fosters a sense of alignment between the body and soul. For the Perfectionist, fasting is not about achieving a perfect cleanse or ticking another box but about embracing the imperfections in the process. It's about honoring her body's need for rest and reconnection.

With this practice, the Perfectionist learns that less can indeed be more. By giving her body and mind the time and space to recalibrate, she gains a deeper sense of self-awareness and strength. This intentional pause allows her to move away from rigid expectations and toward a state of flow, where she can embrace her innate resilience and grace. This healing journey is not just about cleansing the body but also about releasing the emotional and mental patterns that have kept her tied to perfectionism. Through fasting, she begins to rewrite her story with balance, nourishment, and self-compassion.

| FOODS TO AVOID | FOODS TO INCLUDE |
|---|---|
| **Grains:**<br>Buckwheat<br>Corn<br>Millet<br>Rye<br>Yeasted bread | **Grains:** Consume only at lunch, when digestive fire is high<br>Barley<br>Rice<br>Oats<br>Wheat, if tolerated (wheat is often sprayed with glyphosate, an herbicide that can cause leaky gut, among other health challenges) |
| **Vegetables:**<br>Sour vegetables like tomatoes<br>Pungent vegetables like some radishes<br>Garlic<br>Red/purple onions<br>Hot peppers | **Vegetables:**<br>Daikon in moderation<br>Beets in moderation<br>Carrots in moderation<br>Cooked white onions<br>Asparagus<br>Broccoli<br>Brussels sprouts<br>Cabbage<br>Cilantro<br>Cucumber<br>Cauliflower<br>Celery<br>Green beans<br>Leafy greens<br>Mushrooms<br>Okra<br>Peas<br>Parsley<br>Potatoes<br>Sprouts<br>Squashes<br>Zucchini |

| **Fruits:** Avoid sour-tasting fruit<br>Papaya | **Fruits:**<br>Figs<br>Grapes<br>Lemons and limes are fine; though sour, they are cooling in nature as they actually balance heat<br>Apples<br>Apricots<br>Avocados<br>Cherries<br>Coconut<br>Dried fruit<br>Mangoes<br>Melons<br>Nectarines<br>Oranges<br>Peaches<br>Pears<br>Pineapple<br>Plums<br>Pomegranates |
|---|---|
| **Dairy/Fish/Meat:**<br>All seafood<br>Egg yolks | **Dairy/Fish/Meat:**<br>Chicken<br>Turkey<br>Ghee<br>Dairy is normally okay, but for hormonal purposes, we will use it sparingly or completely avoid it. If you use dairy, make sure it is from organic, grass-fed, A2 cows. (The best way to use dairy is by adding coriander and cinnamon and a bit of lemon juice to yogurt.) |
| **Legumes:** Most are well tolerated | **Legumes:** Make sure they are soaked overnight<br>Black lentils<br>Chickpeas<br>Mung beans |
| **Nuts/Seeds/Oils:** Not to consume too much, as they can be too heating | **Nuts/Seeds/Oils:**<br>Coconut<br>Pumpkin seeds<br>Sunflower seeds<br>Flax oil<br>Almond oil<br>Coconut oil<br>Olive oil |

When starting your food plan, take a few days to lay the foundation for detoxing and replenishing. When patients are detoxing and re-establishing new communication with their hormones, I often ask them to give themselves at least three months to allow time for their body and mind to reset. Below is a one-week plan that you can do as a kick start into the three months. This will be a vegetarian-focused week to reset and detox. You will notice that the meals are essentially soup or stew based. This is done on purpose to give your digestive system and your liver a break. You can incorporate some meat in the coming weeks, with at least three vegetarian days in the week.

| DAY 1 | DAY 2 | DAY 3 | DAY 4 | DAY 5 | DAY 6 | DAY 7 |
|---|---|---|---|---|---|---|
| Morning: Green Smoothie (page 199) | Morning: Green Smoothie | Morning: Nettle Mint Tea (page 199) | Morning: Nettle Mint Tea | Morning: Nettle Mint Tea | Morning: Bone broth | Morning: Bone broth |
| Lunch: Borsch, with sauerkraut (page 199) | Lunch: Lentil Coconut Curry, with white basmati rice (page 152) | Lunch: Coconut Smoothie (page 201) | Lunch: Coconut Smoothie | Lunch: Coconut Smoothie | Lunch: Borsch, with sauerkraut | Lunch: Spicy Butternut Squash Soup, with steamed dandelion greens (page 200) |
| Dinner: White Bean and Leek Soup (page 201) | Dinner: Green Soup, with steamed greens | Dinner: Kitchari (page 174) | Dinner: Kitchari | Dinner: Kitchari | Dinner: Lentil Coconut Curry | Dinner: White Bean and Leek Soup, with sauerkraut |

## Nettle Mint Tea

4 cups filtered water
½ cup nettle leaves
½ cup mint leaves
Juice of 1 lemon

Bring the water to a boil. Add the nettle leaves and mint leaves, and boil for 5 minutes. Let steep for another 5 to 10 minutes, then strain and squeeze in some lemon. Enjoy in the morning and throughout the day.

## Green Smoothie

½ cup frozen blueberries
½ banana (previously peeled and frozen) or ½ avocado
1 tablespoon hemp seeds
1 tablespoon cashew butter
1 cup unsweetened coconut milk
1 scoop greens powder

Place all the ingredients in a blender and blend until smooth. Pour into a glass and enjoy!

## Borsch

*4 to 6 servings*

2 tablespoons olive oil
1 medium onion, diced
6 large garlic cloves, roughly chopped
2 stalks celery, chopped
1 cup carrots, sliced small
1 cup diced tomatoes
2 cups beet, thinly sliced
2 cups red cabbage, shredded
½ cup fresh dill, chopped
4½ cups vegetable broth
2 yellow potatoes, chopped
2 tablespoons tomato paste
½ teaspoon allspice
2 teaspoons salt
½ teaspoon pepper
¼ teaspoon cayenne pepper
2 tablespoons apple cider vinegar

Heat a large pot over medium heat. Add the oil and onion, and sauté for a couple of minutes, stirring frequently. Add the garlic, celery, carrots, tomatoes, beet, and cabbage and stir for 5 minutes. Add the vegetable broth, potatoes, tomato paste, and spices and stir. Cook on medium heat for about 20 to 25 minutes, stirring every so often, until the carrots, potatoes, and beets are soft. Remove from heat, add the apple cider vinegar, stir and taste to adjust salt and pepper. To serve, top with fresh dill and enjoy!

## Spicy Butternut Squash Soup

*4 servings*

½ cup raw cashews
2 tablespoons coconut oil
1 small red onion, diced
1 tablespoon minced garlic
6 cups cubed butternut squash, peel removed
1 cup peeled and diced carrots
1 tablespoon minced fresh ginger root
2 tablespoons red curry paste
⅛ teaspoon cayenne pepper
½ teaspoon sea salt
3 cups vegetable broth
½ to 1 cup filtered water

Place the raw cashews in a bowl, cover with boiling water, and set aside for 20 minutes. Heat a large pot over medium heat. Add the oil, red onion, and garlic and sauté for a couple of minutes, stirring frequently. Add the butternut squash, carrots, ginger, red curry paste, cayenne pepper, and salt. Stir to coat. Add the vegetable broth and bring to a boil over medium heat and then reduce to low, cover, and simmer for 15 to 20 minutes until the butternut squash is soft. Let it cool down for 10 minutes before transferring to the blender. Rinse the cashews with fresh water and add to the blender, blend and add the amount of water (up to 1 cup) necessary for desired consistency. Blend until smooth and enjoy!

## Green Soup

*4 servings*

2 tablespoons extra-virgin olive oil
1 large yellow onion, chopped
3 medium zucchini, sliced
1 cup broccoli florets
4 cloves garlic, sliced
¼ teaspoon salt
⅛ teaspoon black pepper
3 cups vegetable broth
1 cup canned coconut milk
½ cup spinach
¼ cup pumpkin seeds

Heat the oil in a pot over medium heat. Add in the onion and sauté for 5 minutes or until soft. Add the zucchini and broccoli and sauté another 5 minutes. Add the garlic, salt, and pepper. Stir. Add the vegetable broth, cover the pot with a lid, turn heat to low, and simmer for 15 minutes. Remove from heat, transfer to the blender, add the coconut milk and spinach, and blend until smooth. Garnish with pumpkin seeds and serve.

## White Bean and Leek Soup

*2 to 3 servings*

1 tablespoon extra-virgin olive oil
½ red onion, finely chopped
3 cloves garlic, finely chopped
3 stalks celery, diced
2 carrots, diced
1 leek, sliced
3 cups filtered water
¼ teaspoon salt
⅛ teaspoon black pepper
2 cups white navy beans
1 tablespoon chopped fresh dill (optional)

Heat the oil in a pot over medium heat. Add the onion and sauté for 2 to 3 minutes until soft. Add the garlic, celery, and carrots, and cook for another minute. Add the leek and cook for another 5 minutes, stirring occasionally. Add the water, season with salt and pepper, and cover the pot to simmer for about 20 minutes until the carrots are soft. Add the beans, cover, and simmer for another 10 minutes. Remove the pot from the heat. Allow it to cool down for 5 to 10 minutes and then blend until you get a smooth texture. Top with dill before serving.

## Coconut Smoothie

*1 serving*

1 cup frozen blueberries
¼ cup unsweetened coconut yogurt
1 teaspoon cinnamon
½ teaspoon nutmeg
2 tablespoon pecans
1 cup unsweetened coconut milk

Place all the ingredients in a blender and blend until smooth. Pour into a glass and enjoy!

## Herbs/Spices: Medicine from the Earth

Herbs and spices are nature's medicine, offering gentle yet powerful support to bring balance back to the body and mind. For the Perfectionist with a Price, these plant allies provide the tools to detoxify, regulate hormones, and create a sense of harmony that has often felt elusive amid her pursuit of doing and being "enough." The herbs for this plan have been carefully selected to address the Perfectionist's specific needs—helping to clear toxins, balance hormonal fluctuations, and calm the nervous system, allowing her to step into a state of greater flow and ease.

Incorporating these herbs into daily rituals—whether through teas, tinctures, or meals—becomes a mindful practice of nourishment and self-care. For the Perfectionist, this is not just about managing symptoms but about reconnecting with herself in a way that honors her needs, her cycles, and her capacity for growth. This approach reminds her that healing is not about perfection but about finding balance, grace, and the courage to trust in the wisdom of her body. Make sure to connect with your practitioner to find the best way to incorporate these into your daily routine.

| NAME OF HERB | ACTIONS |
|---|---|
| Holy basil (tulsi) | An Ayurvedic herb that can help counter physical, metabolic, chemical (even from heavy metals), and psychological stress. Helps your hormonal, immune, and mental health. |
| Milk thistle | Aids in detoxification of excess estrogens from the environment that we come across from beauty products, plastics, and pesticides. It aids in the detoxification process by activation of the cytochrome P450 detox process in the liver. It is protective and restorative and has anti-inflammatory properties. |
| Turmeric (curcumin)—best to use with black pepper to increase its absorption and activate the curcuminoids | Helps to modulate estrogen. Detoxes the liver. Increases the strength of the immune system and is a potent anti-inflammatory. |
| Chaste tree (*Vitex agnus-castus* berry)—can you tell it's one of my favorites! | This herb supports your command center, the pituitary gland, and is progestogenic in nature. Many of the conditions in this plan have an estrogen-dominant nature to them, so this herb is amazing at supporting you! |
| Cleavers (*Galium aparine*) | Magic for the lymphatic system and for painful, swollen, or fibrocystic breasts. Also supportive in clearing your skin due to its draining effects. |
| *Bupleurum falcatum* | Can improve estrogen clearance and detoxification, and correct estrogen dominance, alleviating many PMS symptoms. |
| Triphala ("three fruits": amalaki, haritaki, bibhitaki)—can be taken as a powder in the evening with warm milk (dairy if tolerated, or nondairy) or in a capsule. | Aids in purification of the body and mind, aiding digestion and detoxification. Balances the gut and is a necessary piece in detoxing toxins from the body and rebalancing hormones. By clearing the path in the gut, you clear the communication between the gut and brain, giving your brain more energy and your nervous system the balance it needs to thrive. |

## Vitamins and Minerals

For this plan the focus is to upregulate your detoxification pathways while still supporting your hormones. The below nutrients, along with others from the previous plans, like B vitamins, can help you stabilize your hormones, moods, and other symptoms of estrogen excess and toxicity.

| NAME | ACTIONS |
|---|---|
| DIM (diindolylmethane) | Helps modulate estrogen and estrogen metabolism, allowing the liver to detoxify it out of the body. Caution for those already low in estrogen. It is important to do the DUTCH test to determine whether this would be beneficial for you. It can ease PMS symptoms and help clear your skin. |
| NAD (nicotinamide adenine dinucleotide) | Helps to improve the cells' ability to detoxify and produce energy. One may even see it as the fountain of youth! |
| Calcium D-glucarate | Improves cellular health and estrogen metabolism. |
| Myo- and D-chiro-inositol (combined with alpha lipoic acid) has been shown to improve ovulation and menstrual regulation as well. | Helps to regulate insulin sensitivity and glucose uptake while regulating the menstrual cycle and ovulation. |
| Glutathione | Reduces oxidative stress and inflammation in the body by supporting phase 1 and phase 2 liver detoxification. |
| *Limosilactobacillus reuteri* | One of the most extensively studied bacterial strains for vaginal health, specifically in treating bacterial vaginosis. |
| B complex | Especially needed with any history of birth control use. Needed for most processes in detoxification and hormone support. |
| Binders (zeolite, fulvic acid, charcoal, ethylenediaminetetraacetic acid [EDTA], dimercaptosuccinic acid [DMSA]) | Binders are essential when detoxing to make sure the toxins are getting escorted out of the body. The trick is knowing which one is right for you. For example, EDTA is a more potent binder of lead, while DMSA prefers or has an affinity for mercury. Charcoal and fulvic acid are great for binding on the gut level. |

## Mindset: I Am Enough

When your identity has been intertwined with perfectionism, embracing the concept of surrender can feel both liberating and challenging. Surrendering does not mean giving up or losing control—it means releasing the burdens of toxic thoughts, unrealistic expectations, and limiting beliefs that have kept you striving for an ideal that no longer serves you. For the Perfectionist with a Price, this surrender is not about weakness; it is about reclaiming your inner power by letting go of what has been weighing you down.

The act of surrender works on both the physical and energetic levels, and the breath is one of the most profound tools to facilitate this process. Using the breath as a bridge between the mind and body allows you to clear away the ama—the toxins that have accumulated not just in your physical body but also in your thoughts and emotions. The breath becomes a reminder that your life-force energy is here to nurture and guide you toward your highest good, not the rigid conditions or external expectations that have been imposed upon you.

The Shaman's Breath practice is an ideal tool for the Perfectionist. This breathwork technique helps you tune in to your body, detoxify your mind, and create space for healing and growth. With each inhale, you draw in energy and nourishment, and with each exhale, you release what no longer serves you. This rhythmic cycle mirrors the process of surrender—acknowledging, letting go, and opening yourself to new possibilities.

Through this practice, you allow your nervous system to recalibrate, shifting from a state of tension and control to one of relaxation and trust. Over time, this creates not just a physical detox but an energetic and emotional one, helping you shed the layers of perfectionism that have masked your true self. Surrendering becomes a gateway to authenticity, enabling you to show up in the world as you are—flawed, human, and beautifully whole. This is not just a breath practice; it is a ritual of self-acceptance and empowerment.

*You can sit either in a cross-legged position or on your heels. Interlace your fingers with the pointer fingers pointing out. Straighten your arms behind your back, making sure your palms are together with index fingers pressed together pointing to the earth. Take a few deep breaths in from your nose while expanding your belly and then breathe out through your mouth, bringing the belly back to your spine. Now begin Kapalabhati Breath (Breath of Fire) at a rapid pace for as long as you can and then suspend and hold your breath for as long as you can and exhale. Now contract your perineum/pelvic floor and begin to pulse the energy up into your core. Once you can't do that anymore, move your arms above your head with your pointer fingers pointing straight up to the heavens and repeat the above breath, this time pulsing the energy from above and into your crown, down your spine. Do this for 3 rounds and feel how connected you are to the earth, the heavens, and yourself!*

Note: Kapalabhati Breath, often referred to as the Shining-Skull Breath, is a powerful tool for detoxifying both body and mind. This breathwork practice is like hitting the reset button, clearing the clutter of toxins, stagnant energy, and mental fog. With its rhythmic exhalations through the nose while pumping your navel in and passive inhalations, Kapalabhati creates heat and flow in the body, stimulating digestion, circulation, and your energy centers. It's not just a physical cleanse—it's an energetic one, too, helping you release what no longer serves you so you can step into a clearer, lighter version of yourself.

For the Perfectionist, this practice holds an extra gift. It's an opportunity to let go—of control, of rigidity, of the need to be "just right." Each forceful exhalation becomes a release of the perfectionist tendencies that have kept you stuck, making room for more flow, freedom, and ease in your body and mind. Kapalabhati Breath reminds you of your own power, that within you lies the capacity to transform and shine from the inside out. Try incorporating this into your day, even for just a few minutes, and notice how it invigorates your system and creates space for clarity and calm.

## Morning and Evening Rituals of Bliss

For the Perfectionist, cultivating awareness is a practice of reclaiming balance and grounding amid the constant pursuit of doing and achieving. This process begins with paying attention to how you step into your day and how you release it before surrendering to the dream world at night. It's not just about routines or rituals but about building a conscious connection with yourself—your thoughts, emotions, body, and relationships.

Awareness starts with observing what fuels you and what drains you. Are the thoughts that accompany you through the day uplifting, or are they adding to the pressure you already feel? Does the way you interact with others leave you feeling connected and supported, or does it perpetuate the weight of unmet expectations? For the Perfectionist, it's easy to overlook these subtle signals, because the focus has often been on controlling outcomes or managing appearances. But awareness invites you to shift that focus inward, creating space for reflection and intentionality.

In the morning, this could mean pausing to set an intention that aligns with self-compassion rather than self-criticism. It could mean practicing a mindfulness exercise to check in with your body and recognize its needs. In the evening, this awareness transforms into an act of release—letting go of the tension, the perfectionist narratives, and the to-do lists that no longer serve you. It's about transitioning from doing to being, from striving to accepting.

For the Perfectionist, this journey of awareness is a transformative act of self-care. It teaches you to honor the nuances of your energy, to notice when you need rest instead of pushing through, and to recognize when it's time to step back rather than step forward. By incorporating this mindful awareness, you begin to unlearn the habits of overextension and replace them with practices that nourish your spirit, calm your mind, and support your body. Over time, this gentle shift in focus from perfection to presence can help you move from a state of depletion to one of empowerment.

## Morning

1. Brahmari Pranayama (Humming Bee Breath): Spread your fingers out on both hands and use them to close your ears (with your thumb), eyes (index finger), nostrils (gently with your middle finger), and mouth (ring finger on upper lip and pinkies under the mouth). Inhale deeply. Press the nostril closed and hold your breath for one moment, release the nostrils and hum on the exhale, like there are buzzing bees all around you. Repeat 6 times.
2. Have a color in mind and find 3 objects of that color in your surroundings. This brings you into the moment and into an awareness of the here and now.
3. Stimulate Kapala Marma point: Press the point on your midforehead right by the hairline. This point helps to calm the nervous system and get you ready for the day ahead.
4. Create your declaration for the day. For example, "Today I choose to see my gifts."

## Evening

1. Restorative yoga posture: Lie down on the floor and put your legs up against a wall for 5 minutes. While lying there, breathe long and deep breaths.
2. Say out loud 3 things that brought you joy that day.
3. Take some almond oil and massage your hands, feet, and neck.
4. When lying in bed, repeat 3 times, "I am enough."

## Releasing Control & Cultivating Trust—Relationship Edition

The Perfectionist has built her world around control and careful curation—not just in how she presents herself, but in how she navigates relationships. While she desires deep connection, trusting others feels impossible, and the fear of imperfection keeps her guarded and emotionally distant. Any sign of vulnerability feels like a weakness, and the possibility of rejection is so unbearable that she may push people away before they get too close.

For the Perfectionist, healing relationships means learning to trust, release control, and create safety in imperfection. The tools that follow will help her break free from emotional rigidity, open her heart to connection, and allow relationships to be nourishing rather than exhausting.

---

### 1. "THE LETTING GO EXPERIMENT"—RELEASING THE FEAR OF IMPERFECTION IN RELATIONSHIPS

For the Perfectionist, relationships are often built on performance rather than authenticity. This exercise helps her practice letting go of control in small, manageable ways so she can build trust in others and stop carrying the weight of perfection alone.

**One imperfect action per day**

1. Choose one small thing to do imperfectly in a relationship. (You can start by doing this for one week.) Examples:
    - Send a text without overanalyzing it.
    - Let someone else plan the date night.
    - Ask for help without feeling guilty.
2. Notice the discomfort that arises. Does it trigger anxiety? A fear of being judged?
3. Challenge the thought:
    - "What if imperfection actually deepens my relationships?"
    - "What if I allowed others to see the real me?"
4. Journal about the experience. Did letting go feel freeing or frightening?

**Why it works:**

- Rewires the belief that love is conditional on perfection.
- Teaches the Perfectionist with a Price that relationships can survive (and thrive) without control.
- Allows her to feel supported rather than always in charge.

---

## 2. "THE VULNERABILITY EXCHANGE"—BUILDING EMOTIONAL TRUST IN RELATIONSHIPS

The Perfectionist tends to keep people at a safe emotional distance, fearing that being fully seen will lead to rejection. This practice helps her build trust in relationships through small, intentional acts of vulnerability.

### Couple's Exercise: Sharing Without Fixing *(15 minutes, once a week)*

1. Each partner takes turns sharing one thing they are struggling with.
2. The other partner only listens—no advice, no problem-solving.
3. After sharing, each person reflects:
   - "How did it feel to open up?"
   - "What fears arose?"
   - "Did I feel more connected or more distant?"
4. Practice sitting in the discomfort of being seen.

**Why it works:**

- Helps the Perfectionist trust that love isn't earned—it's given.
- Creates space for emotional intimacy without performance.
- Releases the fear of being "too much" for others.

## 3. "UNMASKING THE MIRROR"— RECOGNIZING HOW PERFECTIONISM AFFECTS RELATIONSHIPS

The Perfectionist often projects her high expectations onto others, leading to disappointment and strained relationships. This exercise helps her identify when perfectionism is interfering with connection and to shift her expectations to embrace imperfection in others.

### Self-Reflection Exercise

### *(use when feeling disconnected or frustrated in relationships)*

1. Identify a recent conflict or frustration in a relationship.
2. Ask yourself:
   - "Am I holding this person to an impossible standard?"
   - "Am I expecting them to show up perfectly so I feel safe?"
   - "What would happen if I gave them the same grace I wish to receive?"
3. Rewrite the story:
   - Instead of "They don't care enough," try "They are doing their best, just like I am."
   - Instead of "They should have known," try "I will communicate what I need."

**Why it works:**

- Shifts the focus from control to compassion.
- Encourages healthier expectations in relationships.
- Helps the Perfectionist with a Price recognize where perfectionism is causing emotional distance.

## 4. "THE TRUST FALL"— REBUILDING EMOTIONAL SAFETY IN A RELATIONSHIP

For the Perfectionist, trust is earned through control and predictability, but real trust requires allowing space for uncertainty and connection. This practice helps her surrender the need for certainty and lean into the unknown in relationships.

### Couple's Exercise: A Physical & Emotional Trust Fall

*(10 minutes, once a week)*

1. Sit across from each other and hold hands.
2. Each partner shares one fear about vulnerability:
   - "I'm afraid that if I open up, you'll think I'm weak."
   - "I struggle to trust that you'll stay if I stop performing."
3. Breathe deeply together for 1 minute.
4. End with a physical trust fall:
   - One partner leans back, the other catches them.
   - Switch roles.
   - Reflect on the experience—was it difficult to trust?

**Why it works:**

- Releases the belief that relationships must be controlled to be safe.
- Creates a deeper sense of security in partnership.
- Allows her to practice trust in both words and actions.

## 5. "PERMISSION TO BE ENOUGH" MEDITATION—RELEASING PERFECTIONISM IN RELATIONSHIPS

The Perfectionist fears that if she is not perfect, lovable, or "on," she will lose connection. This guided meditation helps her release the pressure of performance and feel safe in just being.

### Guided Meditation: "You Are Already Enough"

*(5 minutes before bed)*

1. Close your eyes and take a deep breath.
2. Visualize yourself standing in front of a mirror. Instead of your usual critical gaze, see yourself as someone you deeply love.
3. Imagine whispering to yourself:
   - "You are enough as you are."
   - "You don't have to prove your worth."
   - "You are lovable, not for what you do, but for who you are."
4. As you breathe, allow the words to settle into your body.
5. End with a hand over your heart, repeating: "I give myself permission to be seen, just as I am."

**Why it works:**

- Rewires the belief that love is conditional.
- Encourages self-acceptance in relationships.
- Creates a sense of peace and belonging.

For the Perfectionist, relationships are not about looking flawless—they are about being fully present. Healing is not about becoming perfect—it's about learning that you never had to be.

CHAPTER 12

# Mastering HER—Healing Forward

As women, we are bound by an invisible web of shared experiences, resilience, and innate wisdom. This connection is both our strength and our guide, reminding us that we are never truly alone in our journey. Within this intricate web lies a reflection of the rhythms of Mother Earth herself—her cycles, her creativity, her capacity to nurture and heal. Our bodies carry these same patterns, reminding us of the interconnectedness we share with each other and the world around us.

This final chapter, Mastering HER, is a celebration of that connection and a call to embrace the power we hold within. Throughout this journey, you've explored the layers of yourself—physical, emotional, mental, and spiritual—peeling back the stories and beliefs that have shaped you to uncover the brilliance that has always been there. It's easy to lose sight of our strength in the chaos of life, but remember: Your very existence is a miracle, and your presence is a gift. This is your moment to honor yourself, to fully step into your power, and to claim the space you were always meant to hold. Together, as women, we create ripples of healing, growth, and transformation that reverberate far beyond ourselves. This is what it means to master HER.

## Your Pillars of Mastery

As you apply the tools and insights from this book, it's important to remember that healing isn't a straight line. Even with all the knowledge you now hold, there will still be hard days, old patterns, and moments of doubt. That's why we end with three essential principles—**forgiveness**, **acceptance**, and **devotion**.

These aren't just ideas—they are practices that anchor you as you continue this journey. They are the gentle reminders you return to when things feel messy or overwhelming. When you find yourself slipping into old habits, speaking unkindly to yourself, or expecting perfection, these principles invite you back into connection—with your body, your emotions, your hormones, and your truth.

**Forgiveness** softens the inner critic.

**Acceptance** helps you meet yourself exactly where you are.

**Devotion** is the daily act of choosing yourself with love and commitment.

Together, these practices support everything you've learned through the HER Method and bring it to life—not just as knowledge, but as embodied wisdom. They help you stay rooted in your healing, even when it's hard. Because healing isn't just about what you do; it's about how you show up for yourself through it all.

**Forgiveness** isn't just about making peace with the big, dramatic moments in life—it's about the small, everyday choices to soften your inner world. Most importantly, it's about softening the **inner critic**. That voice—the one that replays your mistakes, questions your worth, and holds you to impossible standards—can quietly wear you down. Over time, that constant internal tension creates stress that affects your nervous system, disrupts your hormones, and distorts the way you see yourself and those around you.

Through this journey, you've learned that forgiveness is not about condoning what hurt you or pretending something didn't matter. It's about **releasing the grip of judgment**, especially the judgment you direct inward. Each time you forgive yourself—for being reactive, for not getting it right, for not knowing then what you know now—you ease that critical voice and make space for healing. You shift from rumination to restoration, from self-blame to self-compassion.

Forgiveness is how you reclaim energy that's been stuck in the past. It allows your body to exhale, your hormones to recalibrate, and your relationships to be met with more compassion and less projection. And perhaps most importantly, it allows you to move forward—not from a place of perfection, but from a place of peace.

Let forgiveness be the practice that quiets the noise inside and reminds you of who you truly are: a woman who is learning, evolving, and worthy of grace. Let it be a daily invitation to soften, to release, and to begin again. This is the path forward—not only in your healing, but in how you live and love from this point on.

**Acceptance** invites us to embrace the full spectrum of who we are—the polarities in our emotions, our thoughts, and our very being. It encourages us to move beyond the binary thinking of "good" or "bad," "success" or "failure," and instead recognize the richness of the shades, colors, and nuances that make up our lives. Acceptance teaches us to honor the days when we feel energized, motivated, and unstoppable, as well as the days when we feel heavy, unmotivated, or overwhelmed. These are all facets of the human experience, all chapters of our story.

Often, our first reaction to feeling "off" is self-judgment—wondering why we aren't as productive, joyful, or resilient as we think we should be. But acceptance reminds us that these fluctuations are not signs of failure but invitations to meet ourselves with compassion. By accepting these aspects of ourselves—especially the ones we've tried to bury or hide out of guilt or shame—we begin to build a bridge to deeper self-understanding. This process helps us integrate the parts of ourselves we've neglected, allowing us to show up fully and authentically.

Acceptance is not about surrendering to powerlessness or resigning ourselves to circumstances we wish to change. It is about recognizing our immense strength to navigate those circumstances, to grow through them, and to reclaim the life that has always been ours to claim. When we lean into acceptance, we stop fighting against ourselves, and instead, we align with the flow of life. This creates space for transformation, resilience, and freedom.

As you reach this stage of your journey, reflect on how far you've come and how much you've uncovered about yourself. Acceptance is a reminder that you are not your struggles, nor your triumphs—these are simply moments within your greater story. Embrace all parts of you, the light and the shadow, and move forward knowing that every piece of your experience has contributed to the unique, powerful, and beautiful person you are. Let acceptance be a foundation as you continue to evolve, making choices from a place of self-love and confidence. It is through this lens of acceptance that you can truly master HER—your hormones, your emotions, your relationships, and yourself.

**Devotion**, an act of radical self-love and one of the most powerful tools for healing and transformation. It is a conscious commitment to yourself, a declaration that your well-being and growth are worth every ounce of effort, time, and care. Devotion requires courage to face the unknown, curiosity to uncover the truths that lie beneath the surface, and the grace to show up for yourself, even when the path feels uncertain. It is through devotion that you create the momentum to move beyond the habits, patterns, and thoughts that no longer serve you.

In this journey, devotion doesn't demand perfection—it asks for consistency and presence. It starts with small, intentional acts of self-care and self-respect. By dedicating yourself to one of the rituals or practices in the previous chapters, you anchor into the daily rhythm of devotion, creating a sacred space for healing and connection. These rituals, no matter how simple, are reminders of your worth, symbols of the love and attention you are giving to yourself.

When you are devoted to your growth, challenges and setbacks no longer feel like failures but rather opportunities for reflection and recalibration. Devotion allows you to pause, to see the lesson in every moment, and to reframe difficulties as part of your evolution. It invites you to approach your healing with flexibility and grace, recognizing that progress is not linear and that every step forward, no matter how small, is significant.

Through devotion, your hormones and emotions are given the space to respond with calm and balance rather than reaction and chaos. Devotion teaches you to pause before responding, creating room for mindfulness in your decisions and actions. This rewiring of old patterns and behaviors shifts you out of survival mode and into a state of thriving. It is in this state that you reclaim your power—power over your health, your relationships, and your life.

Let it remind you that every moment you choose yourself, you are stepping closer to the life you deserve. With devotion, you build a foundation of self-trust, resilience, and joy—a foundation that allows you to master HER, not just as a concept but as a way of being. Devotion is the ultimate act of love and the final bridge to becoming the woman you were always meant to be.

## Returning Home to Yourself

Now that you've connected the dots between your hormones, your emotions, and the way they shape your relationships, you hold the power to change the trajectory of your health and your life. You are no longer at the mercy of circumstance or environment. You've learned how to recognize your patterns, tend to your needs, and make daily choices that support healing and longevity.

Knowing your cycle. Knowing your HERstory. Knowing what nourishes or depletes you. This is your foundation. It's what steadies you when life pulls at your edges. True self-mastery comes not from perfection but from the ability to return to yourself again and again—with clarity, compassion, and choice.

And perhaps the most important choice of all is kindness.

Not just the surface-level kind, but the deep, steady kindness that meets you in your hardest moments. The kind that softens the inner critic. That whispers, "You're doing enough," when the world says otherwise. That sees the patterns of overextending, overachieving, and self-neglect for what they are—survival strategies, not your truth.

Kindness is what allows you to ask not, "What's wrong with me?" but "What do I need right now?"

In the HER Method, this kind of self-kindness isn't a luxury—it's a necessity. Because when your inner world is harsh, your outer world becomes harder to navigate. But when you meet yourself with grace, even in your missteps, you create safety. And from that safety, something profound begins to shift.

Kindness lays the groundwork, but honesty is what carries you forward.

Radical self-honesty means facing not just the truth you tell others, but the truth you may have been avoiding within yourself. It's noticing where you've shrunk to fit in, where you've worn masks to be loved, or where you've silenced your brilliance to keep the peace.

It's also in the smallest choices: choosing to sleep early even if everyone else stays up, to say no when your body says enough, to honor your rhythm even when it's inconvenient. These moments matter. They're how you move from self-abandonment to self-honoring.

And yes—comparison will try to creep in. You'll still be tempted to measure your life against someone else's highlight reel. But you'll know better now. You'll know that every time you look outside for your worth, you leave the present moment—and in doing so, you leave yourself.

This work has taught you to come back.

To stop chasing. To stop fixing. To stop abandoning yourself under the weight of old roles, old patterns, or inherited expectations.

Instead, you now have the tools to choose presence, contentment, and discernment.

Discernment is how you know the difference between a true need and an old habit. It's how you pause before reacting, ask yourself what you really need, and respond with love instead of fear. That pause—that moment of inner listening—is what puts you back in the driver's seat.

From here, healing becomes a relationship, not a race. It becomes less about controlling and more about allowing. You release what no longer serves. You stay open to what's next. You soften into curiosity and let change shape you, rather than resist it.

This is where you return to clarity.

Clarity isn't a single moment. It's a way of living—physically, mentally, emotionally, and spiritually. You've already been practicing it: through the foods you choose, the boundaries you hold, the rituals you've embraced. Clarity clears the noise so you can hear your truth.

And with clarity comes self-discipline—not as punishment, but as devotion. Self-discipline is how you walk your path with consistency, how you honor your body, your needs, and your vision day after day. It's in the little choices, the ones that no one sees but that change everything.

It's in those moments that self-trust is built. That resilience takes root. That transformation begins.

This book has been your companion on the path to self-mastery. And through that mastery, healing becomes inevitable. Because you are no longer just surviving—you are choosing, creating, and living with intention.

To know yourself is to master yourself. And when you do, life reflects that knowing back to you in the form of peace, connection, and joy.

This is the power of HER.

It's not about becoming someone new—it's about returning to who you've always been.

And like the final resting pose in a yoga practice—Savasana—this moment is your invitation to receive. To let it all land. To feel the softness that follows the work. The strength that's been growing inside you all along.

You are here. You are whole. And you are finally home—to yourself.

My hope is that this book has given you permission to dive into the depths of your being so you can unleash the innate power you have. I know life can throw us some curveballs, I know life can feel overwhelming, I know the story you carry has changed so much of who you are, and I also know you are a powerful and sacred woman that deserves a big life filled with all the various textures that life has to offer. So, enjoy this ride of self-discovery and this journey back to yourself as you fall back in love with the most important person in your life, YOU.

# METRIC CONVERSION CHART

| Standard Cup | Fine Powder (e.g., flour) | Grain (e.g., rice) | Granular (e.g., sugar) | Liquid Solids (e.g., butter) | Liquid (e.g., milk) |
|---|---|---|---|---|---|
| 1 | 140 g | 150 g | 190 g | 200 g | 240 ml |
| ¾ | 105 g | 113 g | 143 g | 150 g | 180 ml |
| ⅔ | 93 g | 100 g | 125 g | 133 g | 160 ml |
| ½ | 70 g | 75 g | 95 g | 100 g | 120 ml |
| ⅓ | 47 g | 50 g | 63 g | 67 g | 80 ml |
| ¼ | 35 g | 38 g | 48 g | 50 g | 60 ml |
| ⅛ | 18 g | 19 g | 24 g | 25 g | 30 ml |

**Useful Equivalents for Cooking/Oven Temperatures**

| PROCESS | FAHRENHEIT | CELSIUS | GAS MARK |
|---|---|---|---|
| Freeze Water | 32° F | 0° C | |
| Room Temperature | 68° F | 20° C | |
| Boil Water | 212° F | 100° C | |
| Bake | 325° F | 160° C | 3 |
| | 350° F | 180° C | 4 |
| | 375° F | 190° C | 5 |
| | 400° F | 200° C | 6 |
| | 425° F | 220° C | 7 |
| | 450° F | 230° C | 8 |
| Broil | | | Grill |

**Useful Equivalents for Liquid Ingredients by Volume**

| | | | | | |
|---|---|---|---|---|---|
| ¼ tsp | | | | 1 ml | |
| ½ tsp | | | | 2 ml | |
| 1 tsp | | | | 5 ml | |
| 3 tsp | 1 tbsp | | ½ fl oz | 15 ml | |
| | 2 tbsp | ⅛ cup | 1 fl oz | 30 ml | |
| | 4 tbsp | ¼ cup | 2 fl oz | 60 ml | |
| | 5⅓ tbsp | ⅓ cup | 3 fl oz | 80 ml | |
| | 8 tbsp | ½ cup | 4 fl oz | 120 ml | |
| | 10⅔ tbsp | ⅔ cup | 5 fl oz | 160 ml | |
| | 12 tbsp | ¾ cup | 6 fl oz | 180 ml | |
| | 16 tbsp | 1 cup | 8 fl oz | 240 ml | |
| | 1 pt | 2 cups | 16 fl oz | 480 ml | |
| | 1 qt | 4 cups | 32 fl oz | 960 ml | |
| | | | 33 fl oz | 1000 ml | 1 L |

**Useful Equivalents for Dry Ingredients by Weight**

(To convert ounces to grams, multiply the number of ounces by 30.)

| | | |
|---|---|---|
| 1 oz | 1/16 lb | 30 g |
| 4 oz | ¼ lb | 120 g |
| 8 oz | ½ lb | 240 g |
| 12 oz | ¾ lb | 360 g |
| 16 oz | 1 lb | 480 g |

**Useful Equivalents for Length**

(To convert inches to centimeters, multiply the number of inches by 2.5.)

| | | | | |
|---|---|---|---|---|
| 1 in | | | 2.5 cm | |
| 6 in | ½ ft | | 15 cm | |
| 12 in | 1 ft | | 30 cm | |
| 36 in | 3 ft | 1 yd | 90 cm | |
| 40 in | | | 100 cm | 1 m |

# Bibliography


Acharya, Sourya, and Samarth Shukla. "Mirror Neurons: Enigma of the Metaphysical Modular Brain." *Journal of Natural Science, Biology, and Medicine* 3, no. 2 (July 2012): 118–24. https://pmc.ncbi.nlm.nih.gov/articles/PMC3510904/.

Adele, Deborah. *The Yamas and Niyamas: Exploring Yoga's Ethical Practice.* On-Word Bound Books, 2009.

Andrews, Lia G. *7 Times a Woman: Ancient Wisdom on Health and Beauty for Every Stage of Your Life.* Alcyone Press, 2013.

Babayev, Elnur, and Emre Seli. "Oocyte Mitochondrial Function and Reproduction." *Current Opinion in Obstetrics and Gynecology* 27, no. 3 (June 2015): 175–81. https://doi.org/10.1097/GCO.0000000000000164.

Baird, Donna, and Lauren Wise. "Childhood Abuse and Fibroids." *Epidemiology* 22, no. 1 (January 2011): 15–7. https://doi.org/10.1097/EDE.0b013e3181fe1fbe.

Bastiaansen, J. A. C. J., M. Thioux, and C. Keysers. "Evidence for Mirror Systems in Emotions." *Philosophical Transactions of the Royal Society B: Biological Sciences* 364, no. 1528 (August 27, 2009): 2391–404. https://doi.org/10.1098/rstb.2009.0058.

Behrman, Sophie, and Clair Crockett. "Severe Mental Illness and the Perimenopause." *BJPsych Bulletin* 48, no. 6 (November 13, 2023): 364–70. https://doi.org/10.1192/bjb.2023.89.

Bravo et al. "Ingestion of *Lactobacillus* Strain Regulates Emotional Behavior and Central GABA Receptor Expression in a Mouse via the Vagus Nerve." *Proceedings of the National Academy of Sciences of the United States of America* 108, no. 38 (September 20, 2011): 16050–5. https://doi.org/10.1073/pnas.1102999108.

Brizendine, Louann. *The Female Brain* (10th Anniversary Edition). New York: Harmony, 2007.

Brun et al. "Sex Differences in Brain Structure in Auditory and Cingulate Regions." *NeuroReport* 20, no. 10 (July 1, 2009): 930–5. https://doi.org/10.1097/wnr.0b013e32832c5e65.

Carrasco-Gallardo, C., Leonardo Guzmán, and Ricardo B. Maccioni. "Shilajit: A Natural Phytocomplex with Potential Procognitive Activity." *International Journal of Alzheimer's Disease* (2012): 674142. https://doi.org/10.1155/2012/674142.

Cohen, Marc Maurice. "Tulsi—*Ocimum sanctum*: A Herb for All Reasons." *Journal of Ayurveda and Integrative Medicine* 5, no. 4 (October–December 2014): 251–9. https://doi.org/10.4103/0975-9476.146554.

de Weerth, Carolina, Jan K. Buitelaar, and Roseriet Beijers. "Infant Cortisol and Behavioral Habituation to Weekly Maternal Separations: Links with Maternal Prenatal Cortisol and Psychosocial Stress." *Psychoneuroendocrinology* 38, no. 12, (December 2013): 2863–74. https://doi.org/10.1016/j.psyneuen.2013.07.014.

Diamond, John. *Life Energy: Using the Meridians to Unlock the Hidden Power of Your Emotions.* New York: Dodd, Mead, 1985.

Dornan, James. "The Fall and Rise, of (Some) Women." *Ulster Medical Journal* 81, no. 3 (September 2012): 136–42, https://pmc.ncbi.nlm.nih.gov/articles/PMC3632824/.

Dyer, Cheryl A. "Heavy Metals as Endocrine-Disrupting Chemicals." In *Endocrine-Disrupting Chemicals: From Basic Research to Clinical Practice,* edited by Andrea C. Gore, 111–33. Contemporary Endocrinology. Humana, 2007. https://doi.org/10.1007/1-59745-107-X_5.

Espin et al. "Effects of Sex and Menstrual Cycle Phase on Cardiac Response and alpha-Amylase Levels in Psychosocial Stress." *Biological Psychology* 140 (January 2019): 141–8. https://doi.org/10.1016/j.biopsycho.2018.12.002.

Faleschini et al. "Longitudinal Associations of Psychosocial Stressors with Menopausal Symptoms and Well-Being Among Women in Midlife." *Menopause* 29, no. 11 (November 2022): 1247–53. https://doi.org/10.1097/gme.0000000000002056.

Field, Tiffany, and Miguel Diego. "Vagal Activity, Early Growth and Emotional Development." *Infant Behavior and Development* 31, no. 3 (September 2008): 361–73. https://doi.org/10.1016/j.infbeh.2007.12.008.

Frawley, David, Subhash Ranade, and Avinash Lele. *Ayurveda and Marma Therapy: Energy Points in Yogic Healing*. Lotus, 2003.

Friedman, Michael. *Fundamentals of Naturopathic Endocrinology*. CCNM, 2005.

Fruzzetti et al. "Treatment with D-Chiro-Inositol and Alpha Lipoic Acid in the Management of Polycystic Ovary Syndrome." *Gynecological Endocrinology* 35, no. 6 (2019): 506–10. https://doi.org/10.1080/09513590.2018.1540573.

Garg, Suneela, and Tanu Anand. "Menstruation Related Myths in India: Strategies for Combating It." *Journal of Family Medicine and Primary Care* 4, no. 2 (April–June 2015): 184–6. https://doi.org/10.4103/2249-4863.154627.

Garner et al. "Role of Zinc in Female Reproduction." *Biology of Reproduction* 104, no. 5 (May 2021): 976–94. https://doi.org/10.1093/biolre/ioab023.

Goldstein, Pavel, Irit Weissman-Fogel, and Simone G. Shamay-Tsoory. "The Role of Touch in Regulating Inter-Partner Physiological Coupling During Empathy for Pain." *Scientific Reports* 7, no. 1 (2017): 3252. https://doi.org/10.1038/s41598-017-03627-7.

Gustafson, Craig. "Bruce Lipton, PhD: The Jump from Cell Culture to Consciousness." *Integrative Medicine (Encinitas)* 16, no. 6 (December 2017): 44–50. https://pmc.ncbi.nlm.nih.gov/articles/PMC6438088/.

Harris et al. "Early Life Abuse and Risk of Endometriosis." *Human Reproduction* 33, no. 9 (September 2018): 1657–68. https://doi.org/10.1093/humrep/dey248.

Helfrich-Förster et al. "Women Temporarily Synchronize Their Menstrual Cycles with the Luminance and Gravimetric Cycles of the Moon." *Science Advances* 7, no. 5 (2021): eabe1358. https://doi.org/10.1126/sciadv.abe1358.

Hillcoat, Alexandra, et al. "Trauma and Female Reproductive Health across the Lifecourse: Motivating a Research Agenda for the Future of Women's Health." *Frontiers in Public Health*, vol. 11, 2023, Article 10391316. doi:10.3389/fpubh.2023.10391316.

Hlisníková et al. "Effects and Mechanisms of Phthalates' Action on Reproductive Processes and Reproductive Health: A Literature Review." *International Journal of Environmental Research and Public Health* 17, no. 18 (September 18, 2020): 6811. https://doi.org/10.3390/ijerph17186811.

Holstege, Gert. "How the Emotional Motor System Controls the Pelvic Organs." *Sexual Medicine Reviews* 4, no. 4 (October 2016): 303–28. https://doi.org/10.1016/j.sxmr.2016.04.002.

James, William. "What Is an Emotion?" *Mind* 9, no. 34 (April 1884): 188–205. https://www.jstor.org/stable/2246769.

Kapoor, Amita, Elizabeth Dunn, Alice Kostaki, Marcus H. Andrews, and Stephen G. Matthews. "Fetal Programming of Hypothalamo-Pituitary-Adrenal Function: Prenatal Stress and Glucocorticoids." *Journal of Physiology* 572, pt. 1 (April 2006): 31–44. https://doi.org/10.1113/jphysiol.2006.105254.

Kask et al. "Patients with Premenstrual Dysphoric Disorder Have Increased Startle Response Across Both Cycle Phases and Lower Levels of Prepulse Inhibition During the Late Luteal Phase of the Menstrual Cycle." *Neuropsychopharmacology* 33 (2008): 2283–90. https://doi.org/10.1038/sj.npp.1301599.

Koenig, John. *The Dictionary of Obscure Sorrows*. New York: Simon & Schuster, 2021.

Kok, Bethany E., and Barbara L. Fredrickson. "Upward Spirals of the Heart: Autonomic Flexibility, as Indexed by Vagal Tone, Reciprocally and Prospectively Predicts Positive Emotions and Social Connectedness." *Biological Psychology* 85, no. 3 (December 2010): 432–6. https://doi.org/10.1016/j.biopsycho.2010.09.005.

Kulkarni et al. "The Prevalence of Early Life Trauma in Premenstrual Dysphoric Disorder (PMDD)." *Psychiatry Research* 308 (February 2022): 114381. https://doi.org/10.1016/j.psychres.2021.114381.

Liu et al. "Effects of Endocrine-Disrupting Heavy Metals on Human Health." *Toxics* 11, no. 4 (March 29, 2023): 322. https://doi.org/10.3390/toxics11040322.

Liu et al. "Use of Probiotic Lactobacilli in the Treatment of Vaginal Infections: *In vitro* and *in vivo* Investigations." *Frontiers in Cellular and Infection Microbiology* 13 (2023): 1153894. https://doi.org/10.3389/fcimb.2023.1153894.

Londono Tobon et al. "The Role of Oxytocin in Early Life Adversity and Later Psychopathology: A Review of Preclinical and Clinical Studies." *Current Treatment Options in Psychiatry* 5 (December 2018): 401–15. https://doi.org/10.1007/s40501-018-0158-9.

Malamouli et al. "The Mitochondrial Profile in Women with Polycystic Ovary Syndrome: Impact of Exercise." *Journal of Molecular Endocrinology* 68, no. 3 (March 1, 2022): R11–23. https://doi.org/10.1530/JME-21-0177.

May-Panloup et al. "Low Oocyte Mitochondrial DNA Content in Ovarian Insufficiency." *Human Reproduction* 20, no. 3 (March 1, 2005): 593–7. https://doi.org/10.1093/humrep/deh667.

McGuinn et al. "The Influence of Maternal Anxiety and Cortisol During Pregnancy on Childhood Anxiety Symptoms." *Psychoneuroendocrinology* 139 (May 2022): 105704. https://doi.org/10.1016/j.psyneuen.2022.105704.

Muñoz et al. "Glyphosate Mimics 17β-Estradiol Effects Promoting Estrogen Receptor Alpha Activity in Breast Cancer Cells." *Chemosphere* 313 (February 2023): 137201. https://doi.org/10.1016/j.chemosphere.2022.137201.

Murray, Michael T. "*Glycyrrhiza glabra* (Licorice)." In *Textbook of Natural Medicine*, 5th ed., edited by Joseph E. Pizzorno and Michael T. Murray, 641–7.e3. Eagan, MN: Churchill Livingstone, 2020. https://doi.org/10.1016/B978-0-323-43044-9.00085-6.

Narayan, K. M. Venkat, and Alka M. Kanaya. "Why Are South Asians Prone to Type 2 Diabetes? A Hypothesis Based on Underexplored Pathways." *Diabetologia* 63, no. 6 (March 31, 2020): 1103–9. https://doi.org/10.1007/s00125-020-05132-5.

Pilver et al. "Posttraumatic Stress Disorder and Trauma Characteristics Are Correlates of Premenstrual Dysphoric Disorder." *Archives of Women's Mental Health* 14 (2011): 383–93. https://doi.org/10.1007/s00737-011-0232-4.

Pringle et al. "The Impact of Childhood Maltreatment on Women's Reproductive Health, with a Focus on Symptoms of Polycystic Ovary Syndrome." *Child Abuse and Neglect* 133 (November 2022): 105831. https://doi.org/10.1016/j.chiabu.2022.105831.

Project Viva. https://www.projectviva.org.

Puterman et al. "Anger Is Associated with Increased IL-6 Stress Reactivity in Women, but Only Among Those Low in Social Support." *International Journal of Behavioral Medicine* 21 (2014): 936–45. https://doi.org/10.1007/s12529-013-9368-0.

Raffi, Edwin R., and Marlene P. Freeman. "The Etiology of Premenstrual Dysphoric Disorder: 5 Interwoven Pieces." *Current Psychiatry* 16, no. 9 (September 2017): 20–8. https://womensmentalhealth.org/wp-content/uploads/2017/09/The-Etiology-of-PMDD.pdf.

Rao et al. "Rationale for a Multi-Factorial Approach for the Reversal of Cognitive Decline in Alzheimer's Disease and MCI: A Review." *International Journal of Molecular Sciences* 24, no. 2 (2023): 1659. https://doi.org/10.3390/ijms24021659.

Reilly et al. "The Prevalence of Premenstrual Dysphoric Disorder: Systematic Review and Meta-Analysis." *Journal of Affective Disorders* 349 (March 15, 2024): 534–40. https://doi.org/10.1016/j.jad.2024.01.066.

Rohr, Uwe D. "The Impact of Testosterone Imbalance on Depression and Women's Health." *Maturitas* 41, suppl. 1 (April 15, 2002): S25–46. https://doi.org/10.1016/s0378-5122(02)00013-0.

Ruigrok et al. "A Meta-Analysis of Sex Differences in Human Brain Structure," *Neuroscience and Biobehavioral Reviews* 39, no. 100 (February 2014): 34–50. https://doi.org/10.1016/j.neubiorev.2013.12.004.

ScienceDaily. "'Love Hormone' Is Two-Faced: Oxytocin Strengthens Bad Memories and Can Increase Fear and Anxiety," Science News. July 22, 2013. www.sciencedaily.com/releases/2013/07/130722123206.htm.

Sheffler, Zachary M., Vamsi Reddy, and Leela Sharath Pillarisetty. "Physiology, Neurotransmitters," in *StatPearls* [Internet]. Treasure Island, FL: StatPearls, 2025.

Steegers-Theunissen et al. "Polycystic Ovary Syndrome: A Brain Disorder Characterized by Eating Problems Originating during Puberty and Adolescence." *International Journal of Molecular Sciences* 21, no. 21 (November 3, 2020): 8211. https://doi.org/10.3390/ijms21218211.

Sternberg, Esther M. *The Balance Within: The Science Connecting Health and Emotions*. New York: W.H. Freeman, 2001.

Svoboda, Robert E. *Prakriti: Your Ayurvedic Constitution.* 2nd ed. Twin Lakes, WI: Lotus, 2011.

Sweta et al. "Physio-Anatomical Resemblance of Inferior Hypogastric Plexus with *Muladhara Chakra*: A Cadaveric Study." *Ayu* 38, no. 1–2 (January–June 2017): 7–9. https://doi.org/10.4103/ayu.AYU_140_17.

Towler, Solala. *Tales from the Tao: Inspirational Teachings from the Great Taoist Masters.* China: Fall River Press, 2005.

Veith, Ilza. *The Yellow Emperor's Classic of Internal Medicine*. Berkeley, CA: University of California Press, 2002.

Vineetha et al. "Usefulness of Salivary alpha Amylase as a Biomarker of Chronic Stress and Stress Related Oral Mucosal Changes—A Pilot Study." *Journal of Clinical and Experimental Dentistry* 6, no. 2 (2014): e132–7. https://doi.org/10.4317/jced.51355.

Yang et al. "Association Between Adverse Childhood Experiences and Premenstrual Disorders: A Cross-Sectional Analysis of 11,973 Women." *BMC Medicine* 20, no. 1 (February 21, 2022): 60. https://doi.org/10.1186/s12916-022-02275-7.

Yehuda, Rachel, and Amy Lehrner. "Intergenerational Transmission of Trauma Effects: Putative Role of Epigenetic Mechanisms." *World Psychiatry* 17, no. 3 (October 2018): 243–57. https://doi.org/10.1002/wps.20568.

Zhai et al. "Childhood Trauma Moderates Inhibitory Control and Anterior Cingulate Cortex Activation During Stress." *NeuroImage* 185 (January 15, 2019): 111-8. https://doi.org/10.1016/j.neuroimage.2018.10.049.

Zhang et al. "Onset of Ovulation After Menarche in Girls: A Longitudinal Study." *Journal of Clinical Endocrinology and Metabolism* 93, no. 4 (April 1, 2008): 1186–94. https://doi.org/10.1210/jc.2007-1846.

Zhang et al. "Probiotic *Bifidobacterium lactis* V9 Regulates the Secretion of Sex Hormones in Polycystic Ovary Syndrome Patients Through the Gut-Brain Axis." *mSystems* 4, no. 2 (April 16, 2019): e00017-19. https://doi.org/10.1128/mSystems.00017-19.

Zietlow et al. "Emotional Stress During Pregnancy—Associations with Maternal Anxiety Disorders, Infant Cortisol Reactivity, and Mother-Child Interaction at Pre-School Age." *Frontiers in Psychology* 10 (2019): 2179. https://doi.org/10.3389/fpsyg.2019.02179.

# Index

Page numbers in *italics* reference tables and figures.

# C



# D



# E

## Q



## R

# About the Author

**Dr. Sonya Jensen, ND,** is a naturopathic physician, international speaker, author, and embodied healer who guides women to reclaim their power through hormonal wisdom, emotional depth, and ancestral healing. From her roots in cell biology to her practice alongside her husband, she integrates trauma-informed modalities, herbs, nutrition, longevity medicine, and nervous system support to address the unseen patterns behind hormonal imbalance.

As founder of the HER Method and the HER Community, Sonya helps women decode the stories their bodies are telling—from stress, emotion, and generational trauma—to transform relationships, fertility, perimenopause, and life's transitions. Her work has reached audiences around the world through workshops, retreats, podcasts, and various stages.

**www.drsonyajensen.com**

We hope you enjoyed this Hay House book. If you'd like to receive our online catalog featuring additional information on Hay House books and products, or if you'd like to find out more about the Hay Foundation, please contact:

**Hay House Publishers (India) Pvt Ltd**
Muskaan Complex, Plot No. 3,
B-2, Vasant Kunj, New Delhi 110 070
Phone: +91 11 41761620
www.hayhouse.co.in

—

***Published in the United States by:***
Hay House LLC, P.O. Box 5100, Carlsbad, CA 92018-5100
(760) 31-7695 or (800) 654-5126
www.hayhouse.com® • www.hayfoundation.org

***Published in Australia by:***
Hay House Australia Publishing Pty Ltd
18/36 Ralph St., Alexandria NSW 2015
*Phone:* +61 (02) 9669 4299
www.hayhouse.com.au

***Published in the United Kingdom by:***
Hay House UK Ltd
1st Floor, Crawford Corner,
91–93 Baker Street, London W1U 6QQ
*Phone:* +44 (0)20 3927 7290
www.hayhouse.co.uk

—

## Hay House Titles of Related Interest

*YOU CAN HEAL YOUR LIFE, the movie,*
starring Louise Hay & Friends
(available as an online streaming video)
www.hayhouse.com/louise-movie

*THE SHIFT, the movie,*
starring Dr. Wayne W. Dyer
(available as an online streaming video)
www.hayhouse.com/the-shift-movie

***

*INTENTIONAL HEALTH: Detoxify, Nourish, and Rejuvenate Your Body into Balance*
by Dr. Chiti Parikh

*THE MENOPAUSE RESET: Get Rid of Your Symptoms and Feel Like Your Younger Self Again*
by Dr. Mindy Pelz

*METABOLIC FREEDOM: A 30-Day Guide to Restore Your Metabolism, Heal Hormones & Burn Fat*
by Ben Azadi

*THE PERIMENOPAUSE REVOLUTION: Reclaim Your Hormones, Metabolism & Energy*
by Dr. Mariza Snyder

All of the above are available at your local bookstore,
or may be ordered by contacting Hay House (see next page).

***

*'The gateways to wisdom and knowledge are always open.'*

**Louise Hay**